*The*

# PTSD
# BREAKTHROUGH

THE REVOLUTIONARY, SCIENCE-BASED

## COMPASS RESET
## PROGRAM

# DR. FRANK LAWLIS

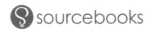
sourcebooks

Published by Sourcebooks, Inc.
P.O. Box 4410, Naperville, Illinois 60567-4410
(630) 961-3900
Fax: (630) 961-2168
www.sourcebooks.com

Library of Congress Cataloging-in-Publication Data

Lawlis, G. Frank.
    The PTSD breakthrough : the revolutionary, science-based compass reset
program / Frank Lawlis.
        p. ; cm.
    Includes bibliographical references and index.
    1. Post-traumatic stress disorder--Treatment. I. Title.
    [DNLM: 1. Stress Disorders, Post-Traumatic--physiopathology. 2.
Stress Disorders, Post-Traumatic--therapy. 3. Psychotherapy--methods.
4. Rehabilitation--methods. WM 172]
    RC552.P67L39 2010
    362.196'8521--dc22
                            2010028216

Printed and bound in the United States of America.
VP 10 9 8 7 6 5 4 3

*Dedicated to the love of our Creator as a vision of taking our next step to paradise, and to the human spirit shown by our troops and their courage on the field and at home.*

# Contents

# Acknowledgments

My first acknowledgment is always to my wife and best friend, Susan, for her love and encouragement to jump in front of the wolves and battle my windmills. She puts up with my dreams and fantasies, and even considers that my ideas might actually work, despite her high intelligence and training in the neurological sciences.

Another friend and constant supporter who most people know as Dr. Phil is on my highest list of acknowledgments. Without his steadfast loyalty and friendship, things never would have worked out the way they have. It is with his support this book was written and endorsed as a major milestone in the treatment of PTSD.

I always wonder why Shannon Marven and Jan Miller, my agents, put up with my projects, because they forfeit a lot of money dealing with my dreams and missions, such as this one. But they do and I am very grateful.

My partner and colleague, Dr. Barbara Peavey, deserves a lot more than she gets for her constant inspiration and brainstorming offered with each project. Between the two of us, we have built our dream clinic where we can see in real time how brain healing does work and the magic of neuroplasticity.

But this manuscript would have never seen much light if it had not been for the early work with Anthony Haskins. Working during those weekend hours in between his life with his new bride, he did his wordsmithing and critiquing with such conviction that I became a passenger on this journey with the book instead of its creator. In addition I want to acknowledge my best sister, Nanciruth Autin, for her ever loving support and loving grammar-fixing.

# Preface

This book is a mission. I am irate about the treatment of our soldiers who come home with a diagnosis of post-traumatic stress disorder, commonly referred to as PTSD. I have witnessed lives destroyed by complete ignorance of the measures that would comfort our soldiers and give them hope for recovery. Even worse, this ignorance is caused by systems blatantly designed to dishonor soldiers and abandon their needs and the needs of their families. (Many foundations have even tried to profit by using their cause for donations.) Some of these systems have been in the press recently; soldiers have been given false diagnoses, such as attention deficit hyperactivity disorder, implying that the problems have been lifelong and not caused by war conditions. By changing the diagnosis, the armed forces are off the hook for liability and insurance coverage.

I am angry about the way the mental health profession,

my own affiliated profession, has brushed off any viable help for people suffering from PTSD. We are supposed to be in an era in which treatment decisions are made on the basis of evidence and results. This is not true in the case of PTSD. Primarily, the decisions on how to handle this disorder are politically based and mired in power struggles. And it's our returning troops who are the victims.

There are many kinds of PTSD, and each case is unique. But as a growing epidemic, the costs of PTSD are high for our country as a whole when we consider the aftermath of this tragedy. By ignoring the seeds of traumatic disorders, we may be paying a higher price in the domestic violence, rapes, bullying, and other forms of violence that some are forced to endure.

Many of us have experienced aggression and even brutality in our lifetimes. The parental abuse statistics are especially troubling, and those statistics only include the cases that have been reported. Is it any concern that, among civilized nations, the United States has the highest rate of violence against children? Elderly abuse is also becoming more common, and we see on the news that armed robbery is being played out in grocery store parking lots and in people's homes. Violence has increased 560 percent since 1960 (www.Leaderu.com). All of this has consequences for our psychological well-being.

What are the answers? Thankfully, there are several important steps that you as an individual can put faith in to prevent and heal this horrible man-made travesty we know and label as PTSD. That is what this book is all about.

Every step in this book is based in science, and the recommendations that follow have brought forth repeated success during four decades of my professional experience. I hope that everyone who treats the victims of PTSD—the war-wounded, military veterans, patients who have been assaulted or injured, and those who have lived through a natural or personal disaster—will read this book and put it to use in their lives.

# CHAPTER ONE

# A New Hope for the Victims of PTSD

Anna knew at her very first glimpse of Richard's face that it was him, and she was elated. As her high-school-sweetheart husband walked through the airport terminal, she was captivated by this moment she had longed for since his deployment months ago. The time had finally come for their long-awaited reunion after his first tour of duty in Iraq.

As she watched him approaching, she waited for his eyes to meet hers—but they didn't. What she saw was not like him at all, and the moment became a confusing event rather than a joyous family reunion after so long apart. Anna watched Richard with his army group as they moved through the small but crowded airport lobby and saw his eyes dart around the space with fear and anxiety, like someone being hunted.

When they finally reunited, there was no soft hug. There

was no meeting of the eyes for reassurance. There was no beautiful moment. Instead, when they embraced it felt like she was holding a stranger in her arms. He bent down and gave what looked like an obligatory acknowledgment of their two boys and then began a swift walk to the car.

Anna hoped that this would be a quick adjustment. She had been warned by the army medical staff that Richard would need some time, so she made a quick decision to show her support by preparing a good, hot supper and allowing him to get a peaceful night's sleep. She was advised that it might take a while until her husband would feel secure in his home again and be able to return to his normal life. She knew better than to expect him to be totally himself on this day. He had just arrived home from fighting in a war, for Pete's sake. But she never anticipated everything that would come.

After just a few hours at home, Richard made a makeshift bed on the floor. A few days later he moved it to the back of their small home. When she asked about it, he quickly and sternly replied that he needed more room and needed to be away from the kids. Anna's heart was breaking. And Richard was showing no signs of improvement. Was this even him? She had never seen him act like this. He was a good husband. A good father. A good man who loved his family.

It was now months since Richard returned from Iraq and

he was increasingly moody and often confused, forgetting even his own children's names. Anna would find him lost within their small three-bedroom house. Many times she would have to direct him to the bathroom, especially at night. He would wander into their bedroom, where she now slept alone, thinking it was the bathroom.

Nighttime was the most difficult. Night after night she lay awake to the sound of Richard crying and calling out in a shrieking voice for whom she assumed were his war buddies. She suspected he was grieving over their deaths. She also heard shouting and screaming as the nightmares victimized his sleep. Anna was witnessing the destruction of her husband's mental capacities on a day-by-day basis. This was agonizing for both of them and was having a profound effect on their two boys as well.

Anna pleaded with Richard to go to the army's medical staff for help, but he refused. He kept telling her that two of his friends were having this same kind of trouble, and when they finally agreed to go to the hospital, they both received the same treatment. When they listed their symptoms and described the gravity of what they were experiencing—extreme moodiness, confusion, terror at night—they were labeled as having "depression" and given medication. It didn't help.

Richard told her that one of these men committed

suicide ten days after he began taking a drug with a warning that read, "Caution: This medication has been shown to have a side effect of increased suicide risk." The other later returned to the hospital again and told the medical staff that he was worse than before. He was labeled as having a "character disorder with impulsive tendencies," and then discharged from the service. They told him that he had these problems before his enlistment. Without much hope of a future after the army, he turned to his own type of medication: alcohol. That brought on a whole new set of problems to haunt him.

Instead of visiting the army medical staff, Richard tried psychotherapy that he secretly paid for out of his own pocket to keep his name confidential from the service. But it did little good. The therapist would try to help him deal with the adjustments of his experiences and fears of the future, but his mind could not focus. After a few minutes, he could barely understand what she was talking about, much less follow her logic-minded ways to find relief from his anxiety or depression. The possibilities of using biofeedback or hypnotherapy were foreign to his background, causing him to become suspicious of such ideas. Even more threatening were ideas like doing yoga or "relaxation therapy." It was like Richard was inside a cloud during these sessions and pretty much everywhere else. It seemed that he was in a separate place observing what was occurring around him—neither here nor there. Trapped inside this misty haze, he felt that at any moment he might explode.

The therapist could have been amazing. She may have been an expert in dealing with the issues of anxiety and depression, but Richard's mind would not allow him more than five minutes' attention in any direction. He could not remember a word said to him by the time he was in his car.

He was encouraged to "talk it out" and be done with it, but that gave him no relief. He felt as if he were only doing these exercises for the curiosity of his therapist. Even though it was explained to him that the horrible events he lived through caused his problems, the memories did not match up with his emotions. The experience was so counter to everything he had ever coped with, and he could not create any psychological mechanism to understand it. He thus tried to block it from his mind and deny the experience, yet the emotional shame and terror remained. He was provided with no magical insight as to why he felt the way he did. He was emotionally dead and scared to death at the same time.

In his regular life Richard wanted peace, but people and social situations only meant irritation and demands. The only way to find relief was to withdraw and drink beer.

In some deep recess of his mind he yearned to be in battle again, to taste the edge of death and smell the gunpowder just so he could feel something, even if it meant feeling intense fear for his life. At least he would know he was alive. He used his favorite revolver to relieve his stress, polishing it daily, not just to keep it oiled and maintained but to touch it and feel its grip in his hand. He would load and cock it, always thinking of the real peace that awaited him if he...

Anna knew what was on his mind, but she had no answers for him. She did not even know this man anymore, this stranger who walked the halls of her house. She was growing increasingly afraid for her children's lives and her own life.

She had good reason. On six different occasions, Richard came into her room screaming with a knife in hand and plunged it into the mattress as she slept. He would barely miss her. At that moment, Richard would awake from his nightmare to find Anna trembling under his hand. He would apologize and withdraw again to his space at the back of the house. Both of them feared that one night the blade would not miss her.

Anna felt as if her life had been spared when the orders finally arrived for Richard to be redeployed for another tour in Iraq. Richard was relieved as well, because he was afraid for his family and what he might do if he had to live like this much longer. As he departed, Anna said good-bye to a stranger, wondering who would return next time.

# What Is PTSD?

This is the story of post-traumatic stress disorder, also called PTSD. The typical term before PTSD was "shell shock," and it was only considered as a weakness in soldiers. PTSD was first considered a disorder when Vietnam War veterans returned with the symptoms listed below, which later became the basis for diagnosis.

The essential feature of PTSD is the development of characteristic symptoms in the senses of the individual following exposure to an extremely traumatic stressor. The stressor usually involves being a part of or witnessing an event of horrific magnitude. The traditional symptoms of PTSD include:

- Nightmares of past traumatic events
- Flashbacks
- Triggers of physical and psychological stresses
- Avoidance of any reminders of similar stimuli
- Isolation from others
- Emotional numbing
- Outbursts of anger or irrational rage
- Problems in concentration and focus
- Hypervigilance for triggers or paranoid thinking

From a rational point of view, all these symptoms seem simple and straightforward, but they are not. There are few treatments that actually show documented benefit in healing PTSD.

Medications for depression and anxiety are usually the frontline treatment. Group therapy has also been a mainline approach, especially with the integration of desensitization techniques. But nothing so far has produced a cure.

## The PTSD Nightmare

There are a daunting number of veterans with PTSD in this nation, with more than eight hundred thousand diagnosed and countless others who have not sought help as thousands of soldiers continue to return home from war. These numbers will cause a seismic shift in our society by the sheer economic cost of care and loss of human capital. This is our national burden, and it's our responsibility to help these men and women.

It's also our responsibility to help the families of these soldiers. The children of veterans with the diagnosis of PTSD are much more likely to have problems in school and trouble with legal boundaries. The experience of having one of your parents become dysfunctional is troublesome enough for a child, but to be emotionally cut off from affection and guidance in understanding your own mixed-up feelings about the world has to be considered as some level of neglect. With spouses suffering from mental health problems, family structures are strained and collapsing at an epidemic rate.

PTSD is not just a problem among our soldiers and their families. PTSD is considered an anxiety reaction to trauma of *any* kind. It can truly happen to anyone.

Luci was brutally raped when she was just fifteen and is still having debilitating nightmares almost every night at age twenty-five. In public, she finds herself hiding from people in closets or nooks, anywhere she can find to feel safe. She is an attractive woman, yet she purposefully dresses poorly to keep men from approaching her. She tries to gorge herself with fattening food to make herself even more unattractive. Therapy is frustrating because she wants to forget the traumatic event, but it seems like the goal of the available therapies is to force her to relive the rape over and over so that she can process her fears about it.

Bill, age fifty-five, was losing sleep because every time he would get comfortable, his doctor's face and voice would invade his consciousness. His mind would immediately go back to the moment he was told he had cancer. When he could finally get some sleep with the help of medication, he would dream of horrible deaths and the nightmares would wake him. He is now afraid of all medical consultations, even those that might help him. He has lost his strong faith in God, feeling betrayed and bitter about these events. He wants to know why this is happening to him. Sometimes, in a fit of anger, he throws things at his wife or lashes out at friends just because they are healthy and happy. With the additional stress caused by PTSD, his immune system is being compromised, which will likely increase his cancer's growth.

Do these people sound like someone you know? Perhaps it is you, your spouse, or a friend. There is a one out of ten chance that you or someone you know will develop PTSD during your lifetime. It's twice as likely if you experience a significant trauma and three to four times as likely if you are involved in some kind of disaster.

It has been shown that the citizens of New York City had a 12.6 percent rate of PTSD due to their close association with the terrorist attack of 9/11. If they were directly involved at any level, the rate shot up to 38 percent. High rates of PTSD are found in professionals who deal with shock, such as trauma counselors, police, firemen, and case workers. And one of the largest populations of people with PTSD is, of course, our soldiers.

The saddest story of all is that, until now, there have been no significant medical approaches to the resolution of PTSD since the diagnosis came into use more than forty years ago. There simply have been no answers. And time is running out.

On average, there are three deaths by suicide each day from veterans alone. More than one thousand attempt to end their lives every month. Although the armed forces count approximately five thousand casualties in recent wars, if you include these suicides and suicide attempts, the number would be closer to seventy thousand.

The two most common treatment approaches for PTSD, medicine and psychotherapy, are not working. Zoloft and Paxil are the only two medications that have been approved by the FDA for treatment of PTSD. But many believe they are contributing to the problem rather than helping it. The labels of these medications warn of a significant risk of suicide. Should we then be surprised that two out of every five veterans who commit suicide were taking these medications? The bottom line: Medication is not the answer.

The other option offered as a solution is psychotherapy. But like Luci, many people with PTSD are not ready to explore painful times again. They are already isolating themselves from their community, friends, and loved ones, so the last thing they want to do is sit in a closed-in office with a stranger for long periods of time. And as strange as it might sound, PTSD isn't cured by exploring feelings or even experiencing reminders of the horrible events that were undergone. These tactics are contradicted in professional psychotherapy because they require the person to relive the painful event in his or her mind without proper preparation or the skill sets to manage the stress that follows.

In spite of the research and poor outcomes, old practices

are hard to change. This approach is not helpful, at least in the beginning, which is where we are right now.

So what is the solution to helping those with PTSD?

## The PTSD Answer

This is where my attitude changes from anger and frustration to excitement and hope. In the past few years I have finally seen the answers that signal the coming of an age when people with PTSD can be helped. I put together the Compass RESET Program for PTSD with the help of Dr. Phil's support, with this new ability to heal PTSD my primary focus. The symbology of a compass is essential to understanding the program. The compass in a PTSD victim has been injured to the point that he or she has become disoriented or confused, misled from within due to trauma and disillusion.

The term *RESET* is the next critical concept, because it is important to start from within to set a new course, one based on the right reasons using techniques that are scientifically based. The term *RESET* stands for the vital mission:

R: Rebooting through
E: Expansion of
S: Strategic and
E: Empowering
T: Therapeutics

The Compass RESET Program gives the individual the clarity of knowing the obstacles that have to be overcome, along with phases required to walk the path to health. A person who has been overwhelmed with trauma cannot be inundated with multitudes of techniques, yet that person needs the assurance of progression and success. The program is designed for those people—created to be relevant for home-based efforts, both for the individual with PTSD as well as the family suffering from its grasp.

I am on a mission to carry the good news to anyone who will listen. (Hopefully that includes not only those in the medical and insurance industries but also the hundreds of thousands of people whose lives have been torn apart by PTSD.) I am not going to give you long, complicated discussions of psychodynamics that no one can understand. I am providing you clear, action-oriented steps based in science that you can take to rid yourself or a loved one of the demons of PTSD.

Recent developments have broken the bonds of traditional treatment boundaries and revealed new paths of healing that produce verifiable results. But no one knows yet—no bulletins have been sent out that have shown the public what is available, what the good news is all about. I don't know why this is, but I'm here to tell you about them.

We now know that PTSD is often the result of a physical

injury to the brain. This happens through a mild or moderate concussive injury, such as a Humvee accident or IED explosion, or being thrown to the ground and hitting your head really hard. But until recent breakthroughs, PTSD has never been recognized as a *biological problem* based in the brain. It has always been regarded as a *psychiatric problem* alone and, as such, could only be treated with psychiatric or psychological methods.

*In order to properly treat PTSD, the biology of the brain must be considered.* As even the armed forces have noted, the new definition and treatments need to include the biological aspects of tissue damage—especially brain injury—and the power of low-risk interventions, such as vitamin supplements and physical exercise. We need to revisit some of the medical approaches that have a less heroic but subtle, effective impact on redeveloping the emotional brain (also known as brain plasticity).

The shift toward a more biological—and scientific—understanding of PTSD is monumental. Psychiatry, which has increasingly been utilized by insurance companies as a vehicle for prescribing medication, has been without much scientific basis for its diagnoses since the birth of the profession, because it was never possible to see the actual psychic damage necessary to clearly define the causality of disorders. Even today, many diagnoses are made purely on a theoretical basis alone, using such guideposts as the strong or weak ego (a mythical structure within the mind). Even the study of chemical interactions in the brain is based largely on rat-brain research generalized to the human brain, and effects are judged on self-reporting of emotional states, which certainly tests the reliability and validity.

I do not say this to condemn the professions of psychiatry or psychology. I only argue that because of the complexity of this disorder, the definition of PTSD needs to be expanded. It can only be treated with an interdisciplinary approach that integrates all of the healing methods we have available. Many of the healing approaches can be done in the confines of your home and are self-directed, which leaves most of the responsibilities for health in the hands of the consumer, not the insurance companies.

It's time for a new definition of treatment for PTSD, one that integrates three essential basics of human healing: biology (healing the brain), psychology (redeveloping the emotional brain), and spirituality (redeveloping the values of the person). Dr. Paul Harch in Louisiana has validated break-throughs through showing that PTSD injures the brain, and it can be healed effectively. There are immediate steps for recovery that can be taken both cognitively and biologically. His research has helped twenty-eight out of twenty-eight military subjects with PTSD to significantly improve their health and be on their way to complete recovery—a 100 percent success rate so far.

Dr. William Duncan should receive a humanitarian award in medicine for his efforts in championing new medical treatments for PTSD, especially for veterans. He has been amazingly successful in getting Congress to act on Public Law 111-5, the Recovery Act, to bring about these breakthroughs on a national scope and requiring insurance companies to honor these new codes. The good news is that several members of Congress, particularly Representatives Walter B. Jones (R-NC), Pete Sessions (R-TX), and Chet Edwards (D-TX), have found out about, believe in, and champion treatments that work. Congress is ready to act on this new solution, and we have the resources *now* to make huge differences.

Now is your time to act, and a new map toward healing from PTSD resides within this book. The solutions prescribed herein are scientific, psychological, spiritual, *and* biological, offering for the first time a fully integrated approach to healing PTSD.

## The Science behind PTSD

This new approach to PTSD results from advances in brain science. With the advent of new technology in the way of brain scans and microneural approaches, we now have unprecedented access to what is going on underneath our skulls. We can harness this new information to better understand

PTSD. Using an electroencephalograph (EEG) to measure the electrical impulses from each area of the brain, I have found the dynamics of PTSD to be very revealing. Without taking you through a course in neuroanatomy, let me just say that for the person suffering from PTSD, the various areas of the brain look similar to this drawing:

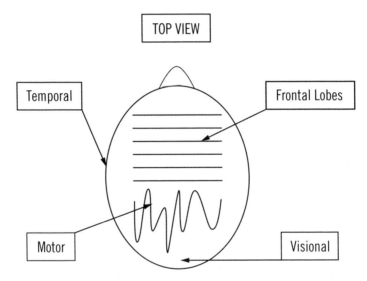

For a PTSD victim, the frontal lobes, which control the executive functioning of the brain (planning and organizing), and the temporal lobes, which handle memory and emotion, are both extremely inactive, almost asleep. Essentially, these areas have shut down. This explains why a person with PTSD commonly experiences no joy and has a very poor memory, little planning or executive power, and poor judgment.

While the front part of the brain is in slowest gear, the motor areas are going haywire. The motor areas of the brain are those associated with coordinating the active parts of our bodies (the limbs, the eyes, etc.). In this state, they are overly reactive. That explains why a person with PTSD might suddenly drop down on his belly or start running when he hears a loud sound similar to gunfire or an explosion. There is also no relaxation and usually no restoration stage in a brain showing this pattern.

Through the study of brain patterns such as these, we have also discovered that there are definite signs of traumatic brain injuries associated with PTSD. Many in the health-care community, including insurance companies and doctors, have been under the assumption that psychological problems were separate from biological problems and did not need the same attention. Those assumptions are no longer true. We now have evidence that PTSD is a complex medical condition, not just an emotional disorder.

Many of those with PTSD have suffered brain damage. The most common form is called *post-concussive syndrome*, which can be caused by direct blows to the head and even heavy sound blasts at a distance. Odd as it may seem, a very loud noise can actually cause mild to moderate brain damage. The strong sound waves continue to cause inflammation in the brain and may cause the immune system to backfire, creating more damage as the signals of cell injury reverberate through the body. Exposure to strong pesticides or heavy metals (such as mercury, tin, and copper), and even some food allergies, can also have a devastating effect on the brain.

## A New Approach to Healing PTSD

Understanding the brain damage behind PTSD opens new approaches to healing. The brain is a remarkable organ, capable of healing itself both physically and psychologically. Once the brain starts the healing process, it can change itself to use new regions and learn to find new avenues for success. New methods of treatment can even help desensitize the brain to the triggers of anxiety and stress.

There are many approaches to PTSD that work with the brain's natural healing process and can be administered by professionals as well as practiced in a person's home. They are inexpensive and straightforward. Surprisingly, many techniques are as old as recorded history itself. For example, the use of special music has extremely powerful influences on the brain. Special foods are available for your home kitchen that will serve your appetite as well as your brain. Certain physical exercises will keep you happier and clear your brain of fogginess and depression.

We also must find and follow our own inner compass toward healing. When PTSD assaults our minds, we often lose that internal direction needed for feeling safe and trusting ourselves. So basic human values have to emerge as the guide to finding hope. Faith may be critical for learning how to find stability and identification. But with these approaches, it is possible for anyone with PTSD to reset his or her own compass and find true north again.

## The Six Steps of Healing PTSD

I have witnessed hundreds of men and women finding the path back to their lives before PTSD by using the Compass RESET steps in this book. Many have also found faith in the sacredness of life again.

But if we want to help ourselves and the ones we love, it must start today. With some simple direction and education, you can stop PTSD from victimizing yourself and others.

This book will help you develop an effective program for healing PTSD. There are seven steps to this program, summarized on the following pages. You will find in-depth information on each step in the subsequent chapters.

### Step One: Nurturing and Healing the Brain

As we have learned, the brain must first be healed of its biological damage before most therapy can take effect. We will examine options such as the hyperbaric chamber, which has proven to be extremely helpful and efficient in healing the brain. We will also discuss the importance of sleep, the primary period in which the brain and body heal. The practice of achieving deeper levels of sleep, which cannot be reached with medication or such substances as alcohol, can be taught and induced with natural approaches. Stress-management techniques specifically for sleep induction can be learned and will last a lifetime. Through associative learning at the brain level and an ordered process of techniques, the individual will learn to sleep at those needed depths to facilitate the healing processes and begin a rebirth of positive thinking patterns.

## Step Two: Cleansing the Brain of Toxins and Poisons

Detoxification of the brain is also a critical process for healing. Toxins and poisons enter our brains due to intentional and unintentional reasons, and unless removed, they can block the next steps of healing from being effective. This chapter covers a wide variety of biological brain detoxification processes that can be done at home or in your physician's office.

## Step Three: Making Reconnections and Taking Control of the Disoriented Brain

Too often, psychology-based programs attempt to change a particular thought pattern to heal PTSD, using hypnosis or reinforcement procedures, but they ignore the rest of the brain. These methods quickly fail. In this chapter, I will offer a new approach that digs deeper and fully integrates the brain, uncovering the central self who is in charge of thoughts and has to be consistent with who we are if we are to heal ourselves. Through this problem-solving approach, we find personal resolution through individual creativity and gains of self-confidence. It is finding peace in challenges. This step is accomplished by creating multisensory communication networks using sound, voice, visualizations, and touch and body movements. It also includes self-confidence builders and other exercises to enhance self-authenticity and strengths.

The major complaint of individuals suffering from PTSD is lack of control. They can't stop the thoughts of traumatic experiences, the nightmares, and usually can't stop feelings of emotional pain. They are in what I call "stress storms" at the brain level, and they feel trapped. They feel they are "going crazy" and often report demons entering and controlling their minds. Although irrational in nature, these reports make perfect sense when we view the brain scans of these individuals.

Often, when the brain is vulnerable to destructive thoughts and unable to cope, there is a tendency for the person to use self-dialogue learned from frustrating challenges. For example, there are often memories that reflect defeating messages from significant others, like a father saying, "You will never amount to anything. You are as useless as a knob on a tree. You will never amount to anything." Messages are then internalized and remembered at times in which self-confidence is at its lowest, and they become entwined in the stress of the present. Guilt, depression, anger, and other emotions can create a trap that only decreases a person's mood and self-confidence. These negative internal conversations have to be confronted and dismantled.

The individual must learn to "cleanse" himself of this emotional baggage. There are inexpensive devices and special techniques available to facilitate the process and help rid the anxieties and fears from the mind.

## *Step Four: Relinquishing Fear and Rage*

What we know about brain function is that problem solving and proactive planning is centered largely in the frontal lobe of the brain, and it sometimes has to be jump-started to find solutions. This can be accomplished with positive-thinking coaching, power breathing, posturing with rhythmic balance, exposure to blue light, reconstructing positive-memory selection, and even chewing gum. It is important to learn how to energize the mind with self-nurturance. Techniques from ancient medicine and traditional principles are brought forth and can help create a life plan to earn the joy and accept the honor and privilege of life. Through correct brain stimulation into the joy centers, the spirit of life can find optimistic hope for the future.

## *Step Five: Creating a New Beginning*

Regardless of a person's culture or beliefs, the brain has to be open to the paths of basic spiritual needs, which can include a sense of higher purpose or a set of core values.

The steps that are important to rediscover this realm of personal connection are:

• To accept and receive love

• To feel the safety within that realm of reality

• To be open to being a part of something greater than yourself

## *Step Six: Reestablishing Your Internal Compass*

This final step focuses on reentering the community. When a person has been traumatized, there is often a sense of betrayal that has to be overcome, even though the trauma may not have been anyone's fault. It may be a state of loneliness in which the person feels that no one understands the emotional upheaval that has taken place, leaving them isolated. Fear and anxiety can manifest on both sides of a relationship. The individual has to learn how and whom to trust and develop a sensitivity to behaviors of withdrawal and hostility.

There are several different approaches that are effective at home or in a sanctuary. Some people find that PTSD can actually serve as a springboard to higher realizations and skills. Regardless of how it is received, it is imperative for the effort to be made to fully regain one's soul.

## The Time Is Now and It Is Urgent

I only regret that this book may have come too late for many people whose lives were lost to the desperation of PTSD and for the families who witnessed the defeat of a human soul. But thankfully, we can now prevent this from happening.

My hope is that with this book as a guide, PTSD will become only a memory for its victims, and the battle will become another step toward understanding the bountiful power of our minds, the full extent of which is still not fully known.

# Chapter Two

# Step One: Nurturing and Healing the Brain

As we have learned, PTSD often includes biological damage to the brain along with the psychological trauma. Thus, in order to truly heal PTSD, the first step is to heal the damage done to the brain. This chapter will focus on the cornerstones of brain healing:

- Hyperbaric chamber treatment
- Vitamins and minerals
- Sleep

## Do You Have Brain Damage?

Before you can reboot a computer, you must first correct any problems that exist. Otherwise, it will just crash as before. The first step in the RESET program is the same. You must assess whether brain damage has indeed occurred. If you know that you have sustained damage to your brain, skip ahead to the next section and learn about your brain-healing options, the first step for PTSD recovery. If you're not sure, consider doing the following exercises to see if you have any of the symptoms.

NOTE: There are several ways to determine if someone has sustained damage to his or her brain, but it takes a professional neurological examiner to fully assess this question. These are simple tests to try at home, and should not be used as a diagnosis but rather as a first step in understanding the extent of your PTSD.

The following are a few methods that are very similar to the way of measuring brain-related cognitive problems. The first is called the Memory Sample Assessment. You will need someone to help you with this assessment, though it is very simple and can be conducted by just about anyone. Have him or her read aloud a random sequence of letters, starting with just two letters and increasing the length from there. Then repeat them back in a slow and consistent manner. For example:

F – X
S – Y – T
G – N – W – P

J – L – V – Z – Q
U – B – H – D – P – W
C – W – K – B – G – X - Q

The average person can remember five or more letters. If you are not able to list five or more, it may mean you have biological brain damage.

Next is a verbal exercise. Begin the same way, but this time repeat the letters backward. So if the person said F-G-I, you would say L-G-F to get it right.

X - F
T – Y – D
P – W – N - G
Q – Z – V – L - J
W – P – D – H – B - U
Q – X – G – B – K – W – C

As you can see, this exercise requires more memory because you have to remember the letters and turn them around. Most people can get four letters in this exercise. If you cannot get four or more letters, once again, it may mean there is biological brain damage.

Do this visual test in a similar fashion, but this time use symbols. First, study each line of symbols. Next, hide the symbols. Then try to redraw the symbols in the correct order on a separate piece of paper.

Here are the lines of random symbols you might use:

Line 1: ⌂    ∩
Line 2: ☐    ♂    ☼
Line 3: ☺    ⌂    ♦    ♀
Line 4: ▼    ◊    ○    ♥    ▫
Line 5: ∩    ▲    ♠    ◊    ☼    ᅲ

Studies show that most people can remember and redraw five symbols. If you cannot remember five or more, it may mean that there is biological damage to the brain.

Here are some additional tests that are often used to determine brain damage and trauma.

## 1. Find the C below:

OOOOOOOOOOOOOOOOOOOOOOOOOOOOOOO
OOOOOOOOOOOOOOOOOOOOOOOOOOOOOOO
OOOOOOOOOOOOOOOOOOOOOOOOOOOOOOO
OOOOOOOOOOOOOOOOOOOOOOOOOOOOOOO
OOOOOOOOOOOOOOOOOOOOOOOOOOOOOOO
OOOOOOOOOOOOOOOOOOOOOOOOOOOOOOO
OOOOOOOOOOOOOOOOOOCOOOOOOOOO
OOOOOOOOOOOOOOOOOOOOOOOOOOOOOOO

OOOOOOOOOOOOOOOOOOOOOOOOOOOOOOOO
OOOOOOOOOOOOOOOOOOOOOOOOOOOOOOOO
OOOOOOOOOOOOOOOOOOOOOOOOOOOOOOOO

**2. Find the 6 below:**

9999999999999999999999999999999999999999999
9999999999999999999999999999999999999999999
9999999999999999999999999999999999999999999
6999999999999999999999999999999999999999999
9999999999999999999999999999999999999999999
9999999999999999999999999999999999999999999

**3. Find the N below:**

MMMMMMMMMMMMMMMMMMMMMMMMMMMMNMM
MMMMMMMMMMMMMMMMMMMMMMMMMMMMMMMM
MMMMMMMMMMMMMMMMMMMMMMMMMMMMMMMM
MMMMMMMMMMMMMMMMMMMMMMMMMMMMMMMM
MMMMMMMMMMMMMMMMMMMMMMMMMMMMMMMM

To find the figures requires some concentration, and it is generally agreed that most people can find at least two of them.

There are also some general ways to test for critical thinking skills. This test involves solving a problem in which there is a need to think out the solution in a logical manner. Some examples are listed below:

- How old is Sam if he is five years older than Judy and Judy is four years older than Jim and Jim is two years old? (Answer: Eleven)

- How much change would Sam get back if he had $10.00 and bought five peaches at fifty cents apiece and two candy bars for $1.50 a piece with a drink costing two dollars? (Answer: $2.50)

- What is the least number of trips (counting each way across as one trip) it would take to get seven people across a river if you had a raft that only carried four people and it takes two people to paddle it? (Answer: Five)

Coming up with the correct answer is not as important as assessing if the steps taken for solving each problem were logical, reasonable, and had some purpose. You can do this by verbalizing each step in the thinking process. These kinds of problems also double as tests for attention and concentration.

If your assessment shows that you have sustained brain damage, it is time to begin the road to recovery. The first cornerstone of brain healing is using the hyperbaric chamber treatment.

# 1. The Hyperbaric Experience

The hyperbaric chamber treatment can revitalize portions of the biologically damaged brain and is one of the most effective treatments for PTSD. The simplest way to explain what the hyperbaric chamber does for you is that it uses pressure to infuse a high concentration of oxygen into your body. With this high level of oxygenation, the healing rate is drastically increased. This is true whether it is sores on your feet or damaged portions of the brain. To some, it may not sound like real medicine because it does not hurt, and technicians don't prod you or stick gauze in your mouth. But it is a very powerful tool in regenerating damaged areas of the brain.

The hyperbaric chamber treatment is the best way we have found to get the brain on the healing track. For most it is a very positive experience, regardless of outcome. There are no medications that make you goofy, no surgery on your brain like a lobotomy, no electric shocks, no shots, no pain, and no uncomfortable or embarrassing positions to deal with. It's simple and easy.

You change into pajamas or other comfortable clothes. Then you climb into a soft, relaxing bed that is placed inside a metal container that from the outside looks like a large, shiny barrel. There is no threat of claustrophobia because you have a large, curved window through which you can speak to people on the other side and therefore do not feel isolated.

You can have music of your choice playing inside, but some people just like to sleep. Once inside, you lie in complete rest for about forty minutes (depending on the treatment plan). After your session is over, you leave. Most people describe the experience as being the most relaxed they have felt in a long, long time. A typical treatment plan includes forty or more of these sessions.

During the course of your hyperbaric treatment, the oxygen pressure is increased to about one and a half times the air pressure outside the chamber. It doesn't feel much different than normal because the air pressure increases gradually. In the beginning, you don't feel too different, mainly because the brain is being repaired at levels below your consciousness by the pressurized oxygen on your tissues. Sometimes at about the twentieth session, you might feel strange or agitated and worry that you are changing in ways you do not understand. You are changing, but only in positive ways. It usually means your brain is making you aware of the constructive process and encouraging you to relax and get some sleep. These are very beneficial results on all levels, especially in the treatment of PTSD.

Your body does its best healing when you are asleep or very relaxed, because the immune system is allowed to work at its best during those times. Your system of internal healing is based on the state when you are not being stressed and pressed, which is the reason you are most vulnerable to illness during prolonged periods of anxiety or depression. During the continuation of your hyperbaric chamber experience, there are usually a long series of deep sleep periods during which you are gaining huge strides toward a more complete biological and psychological health.

From a patient's point of view, the hyperbaric treatment experience is more like a spa treatment than a medical one. But it is most critical step in the healing process of PTSD. There are highly trained specialists who monitor you and your vital signs during the treatment, so all you have to do is kick back and leave everything to the medical team. And to think, this is the beginning, and everything gets even better from here.

Hyperbaric treatment is getting easier to find as insurance companies are more willing to support its use. Since its use rarely has medical complications, there has been low resistance to referrals to hyperbaric centers, although very little encouragement has been noted. It may still be categorized as an "alternative" treatment with the connotation of being a "fad" medicine.

## JAMES'S STORY

Before beginning a hyperbaric chamber trial, James's neurological cognitive abilities were tested to see if he might have biological damage. It was hardly surprising from his wife's description of his problems that the results showed he was very affected at the level of brain functioning. His memory, abilities to organize his thoughts and pay attention, and overall intelligence were all barely on the performance of a third grader, even though he had received a college degree. He often lost his way home when going out for errands, and usually forgot the reason for his errands once he was out and about. He had difficulty trying to read or make sense of the news of the day or discussing any aspect of his family's problem-solving challenges, such as how to help with child care (his wife didn't allow him to supervise their young children by himself) or even deciding when to eat (he would react impulsively to his hunger regardless of the time of day).

At the clinic, he signed up for forty hyperbaric chamber sessions (one per day). Although the progress was slow for about three weeks, by the end of his forty days, he showed amazing results. He continued his treatment for twenty more sessions, and at the end of that process, he was tested again. His memory and abilities to organize thoughts and material began showing levels of functioning above the national average, and his intelligence score (IQ) soared thirty points.

James was now becoming excited about life again. Both he and his wife reported no further problems at home. This brought peace for him on a personal level as well as on a social level with both friends and family. He had regained his self-confidence and was ready to return to the navy, which he did right away. If you calculated the cost/benefit savings to the government for the rehabilitation of James, for just this short period of time, the navy saved over $155,000 by simply integrating the hyperbaric chamber in the treatment of his PTSD.

James is one of the fortunate patients who only needed the hyperbaric chamber treatment to jump back into his everyday life. While he may be an exception to the general practice, research has shown that you can predict that the treatment will provide at least 40 percent of the solution to healing your PTSD. And as the initial process for the healing portion of the brain in the treatment of PTSD, it is 100 percent part of the critical stage of healing.

## 2. Vitamins and Minerals to Nurture Your Brain

The second cornerstone of brain healing is the proper intake of vitamins and minerals. To help an injured brain get better faster, it is essential to give it good nutrients in the form of vitamins and minerals, but you must choose them carefully. A recent study that examined the nutritional quality of supplements in different vitamin and mineral products found that one-third of the products contained no presence of the ingredient being advertised, and another third showed only minor amounts. Only one-third contained enough of the advertised substances to be considered therapeutic. In this chapter I will recommend several of the best supplements, but you should also use your judgment as to which you think would be most helpful for you. When purchasing them, insist on pharmaceutical-quality ingredients and recommended health-food brands, which can be purchased at most drug stores.

## Omega-3 Fatty Acids

At the front line of the brain healing process is *neurogenesis*, the rebirthing of nerve cells. Research shows that omega-3 fatty acids, which are abundant in certain fish and plant foods, can aid in this regeneration of brain cells. Omega-3 fatty acids help insulate the neurons in the brain, which increases the speed of nerve impulses and connections, thereby increasing the rate of healing at the biological level. They are also known to combat depression, enhance learning and memory, and serve as major aids to brain plasticity (creating new neuropathways needed for constructive changes in the brain).

Omega-3 fatty acids are found mostly in plant foods such as flax, soybeans, and vegetables. They are also found in fish; just a four-ounce portion of salmon twice a week serves about five grams of omega-3, which is the amount recommended for brain food.

Not all fish produce the same quantities of omega-3 fatty acids, as you can see in this table:

## Omega-3 in Fish per Ounce

| | |
|---|---|
| Sardines | 3.3 g |
| Mackerel | 2.5 g |
| Salmon | 1.8 g |
| Herring | 1.7 g |
| Bluefin tuna | 1.6 g |
| Lake trout | 1.6 g |

## *Thiamine (Vitamin B₁)*

This substance helps manufacture acetylcholine, one of the brain's major messengers known as neurotransmitters. It triggers the metabolic process that helps the brain better use the food available to it. Even if you consume high amounts of fish, if you don't get a little $B_1$, there is little chance of improvement in brain health. The very best place to find vitamin $B_1$ is in nuts and grains.

## *Vitamin D*

This is the sunshine vitamin (named for its development in the skin when exposed to the sun), which is vital to the brain and has been considered as a possible factor in fending off Alzheimer's disease. Vitamin D is critical in maintaining the ratio of calcium and phosphorus, critical to promotion of growth for nerve cells. Vitamin D has also been reported as a major helper of the hippocampus, the primary memory control center of the brain, and it is therefore very effective in the healing process of brain injury.

## Strategic Nutritional Plan for Memory

Since memory is an intellectual function that is integrated with other processes, memory loss is usually associated with many kinds of brain injury. Memory is critical for learning and storing new information to help you overcome the unique challenges of each day, and thus is essential to the process of recovering from PTSD. If you are experiencing memory problems, these must be corrected. Below is a list of supplements that can help improve your memory retention.

- **Acetyl-L-carnitine (dosage up to 1,000 mg a day)** has been shown to promote the activity of two neurotransmitters, acetylcholine and dopamine, both of which improve the communication among the parts of the brain, which enhances creativity and higher-level problem solving, reflex speed, and efficiency.

- **Alpha-glycerylphosphosphorylcholine (Alpha-GPC) (400 mg three times daily)** is rich in choline, the major ingredient in chicken eggs that has been shown to raise IQ scores. It combines glycerol and phosphate, which protects the brain cell membranes, thereby producing better memory. It also appears to have amazing recuperative properties for stroke patients in the areas of intellectual functioning, making it a major candidate for other brain injuries as well.

- **Choline (1,500 mg daily)** is widely applauded as a mental stimulant that makes you smarter. It is produced within your body from two amino acids, methionine and serine, with help from vitamin $B_{12}$ and folic acid.

- **Ginseng (follow dosage on bottle)** gets a lot of attention for promoting good health and mental alertness, but it can also be quite corrupted in quality. There are reports of some unethical suppliers out there. Ginseng contains ginsenosides, which stimulate the brain's neurotransmitters so that it can synthesize proteins optimally for brain fuel. Many studies have found evidence of its power to stimulate mental capacities.

- **Rhodiola (follow dosage on bottle)** is a Siberian herb that soldiers have used for stamina and has shown excellent results in mental states, especially depression. I have seen it help patients improve more quickly from a series of brain complications, but there are no studies readily available to show the actions it takes on the cellular level.

# 3. Sleep: The Master Healer

The third cornerstone of brain healing is found in the power of sleep. Sleep is the best way for your mind and body to recover from any problem. Unfortunately, lack of sleep or the ability to experience peaceful sleep is one of the biggest problems people suffering from PTSD must deal with. This is because the PTSD brain has been tormented and programmed only to survive.

What does this mean? Imagine that the human brain functions the same way a dolphin's does. The dolphin has to breathe to stay alive, but it also has to sleep. The dolphin has found a way to have half its brain go to sleep while the other half stays awake and maintains the cycle of surfacing to breathe. Occasionally the dolphin switches sides so that it can complete restoration of both sides of the brain uniformly.

The human brain is not engineered this way, but it does act in a similar way when the brain is constantly geared toward fear. When someone is suffering from PTSD, their mind is always alert to the threat of harm or pain. Thus, even when performing normal functions of the day, part of the brain is always alert and on the lookout for danger. And it even does this while the PTSD victim is sleeping.

The result of this very creative way of the brain to stay alive is poor sleep. And human beings don't work well over a long period of time without restful sleep. Your body and mind become exhausted. In order to fully function, you must experience each of the five stages of sleep each night:

- **Stage 1**: This is the time when you fall asleep and is a transition stage that occupies approximately 2–5 percent of a normal night of sleep. For people with insomnia, this stage lasts much longer and prevents deeper rest.

- **Stage 2**: This stage occupies approximately 45–60 percent of sleep. You are generally considered at the door of restoration cycles and go on a type of roller coaster of levels during this stage that have a variety of important effects on the healing process.

- **Stages 3 and 4**: This stage is often referred to as delta sleep. Contrary to popular belief, it is this delta sleep that is the "deepest" stage of sleep (not REM) and is what a sleep-deprived person's brain craves the most. In adults, it can last from fifteen to thirty minutes. In children, it can occupy up to 40 percent of all sleep time (this is why it seems impossible to wake children during most of the night).

- **Stage 5:** Rapid eye movement (REM) sleep is an active stage that composes 20–25 percent of a normal night's sleep and is when vivid dreams can occur. It is called rapid eye movement sleep because if one watches a person in this stage, the eyes are visibly moving rapidly under the eyelids. After the REM stage, the body usually returns to stage 2 sleep. You can have many cycles through REM sleep.

Understanding these stages is important because our psychological and physical restoration is affected differently in each stage. For example, other than losing alertness, not much happens in stage 1. It is in later stages that you start to gain physical restoration. In the even deeper stages of delta and especially REM sleep, your brain has the ability to find resolutions to its built-up stresses.

Sleep-deprived individuals experience problems because sleep medication and most sleep aids, especially alcohol, can only assist you in achieving stage 1 sleep. This light stage of sleep really doesn't help you much, and further, many sleep-enhancing drugs can become addictive. What's more, PTSD patients often experience fear of the loss of control required for deep sleep and lack the skills to release into these deeper levels.

Therefore, it is crucial for PTSD victims to learn to recover the ability to sleep well and deeply again. Although there may be many challenges for the person with PTSD to achieve a good night's sleep, there are several easy-to-follow sleep techniques that will help in beginning the journey toward a more complete and restful sleep.

## Sleep Management Skills

Sleep cycles must be mastered in order to reach the maximum benefit of the restoration therapy that deep sleep provides to both the body and the mind. The following techniques are a guide for the beginning, middle, and end of your path toward complete healing and for continuing health.

### *Circadian Rhythms*

We all possess a biological clock, known as our circadian rhythm, which dictates the rest period for our minds and bodies in every twenty-four-hour period. An internal biological clock is fundamental to all living organisms, influencing the release of hormones that play a vital role in sleep as well as wakefulness, metabolic rate, and body temperature. Each of us is different in our circadian rhythms, and if you neglect these important cycles, you pay the price through fatigue, pain, stress, and, in some cases, even death.

A good example of how we are all governed by our circadian cycles is jet lag. Anyone who has traveled cross-country via airplane has surely experienced this groggy feeling associated with beginning the day in one time zone and ending it in another. We also allow our environment to disrupt our circadian patterns when we watch television or surf the Internet until the early morning hours, or when we extend poor eating and drinking habits into those periods of restoration. Alcohol and sugar have both been documented as negatively affecting circadian cycles.

If you compound the common problems of circadian effects with the problems of a person with PTSD, along with the challenge of relaxing and the counter-productive effects of prescription medications and/or self-medication (drugs and alcohol), you see the problems that arise. And you can see just how important it is to get deep, restorative sleep. The good news is that it's possible to change your lifestyle to achieve harmony with your natural circadian cycles, and in doing this you will experience success in effective sleep patterns. A step-by-step plan for realizing this much-needed quality sleep is listed below.

**Step One: Awareness**

The first step is simply to become aware of your own circadian rhythm. You can do this quite easily by identifying the times of day you consistently feel the most effective and useful. As you do this, note the kinds of things you like to do during these times. Also note times you feel the least active and focused, and what you like to do during these times.

6:00–8:00 a.m. _____

8:00–10:00 a.m. _____

10:00 a.m.–noon _____

12:00–2:00 p.m. _____

2:00–4:00 p.m. _____

4:00–6:00 p.m. _____

6:00–8:00 p.m. _____

8:00–10:00 p.m. _____

10:00 p.m.–midnight _____

12:00–2:00 a.m. _____

2:00–4:00 a.m. _____

4:00–6:00 a.m. _____

**Step Two: Acknowledge Needed Changes**

Make a note of the kinds of activities you do in order to modify your circadian rhythm to feel more awake or more relaxed, such as drinking too much coffee, taking stimulants, consuming alcohol, taking sedatives, doing physical exercises, eating food, etc. Indicate how well these work for this purpose. Find out for yourself what elements contribute to or take away from your ability to achieve harmony with your natural circadian rhythm. Also note what kinds of activities might be explored to improve this harmony (nutrition, relaxation, etc.). One good way to do this is to keep a diary or journal of how naturally you go through your cycles and the activities or foods that might influence how well you feel.

**Step Three: De-stress Your Sleep**

Stresses, especially fear and anxiety, are major hindrances to the effective quality of restorative sleep. When you experience stress, there is a biochemical reaction that occurs in the brain that alerts you in the same way it does when there is a fear response. Hence, the brain goes into protection mode. The hormones are alerted and a call to action is sent to those systems we use in emergencies. Your body produces a higher heart rate, higher muscle tension, more adrenaline flow for energy, and a host of other reactions, all of which are diametrically opposed to achieving a deep restorative sleep state. Stress therefore inhibits biochemical readiness for sleep. So how do you prevent this damaging stress from invading your much-needed restorative sleep?

One of the easiest ways to de-stress your sleep is to "teach" your mind how to go sleep. There are some very good sleep CDs that use rhythms and melodies with step-by-step instructions to guide your mind and body into the deeper sleep zones. By not having to mentally focus your mind on the steps of relaxation and distraction strategies, you can allow your mind to enter the sleep zones easily. This inexpensive and easy tool can teach your brain to find the pathway to a more restorative sleep. The brain does so in stages. These stages are achieved on their own without any participation from you. Simply lie down in a comfortable position, put the CD in, and let it do the work. I have found the sleep series CDs at www.MindBodySeries.com to be particularly useful. You can feel confident in their success as a tool to bring relief from sleep deprivation, as well as a host of other mind-body issues.

By allowing your brain to learn by listening without judgment or criticism of yourself or the CD, you may find long-term success. Eventually all you'll have to do is start the process and your mind will do the rest automatically. The CD literally teaches your brain how to go to sleep. There is a script for this that I recommend, which can be found in the appendix of this book.

**Step Four: Rumination Control for Restorative Sleep**

The next step involves simplifying your brain so that you can reach peaceful restorative sleep. Contrary to what many people think, the most frequent disturbance affecting sleep patterns is not outside noise, but rather the noise coming from within the mind. Often, it's the panic of your mind trying to solve all your worries twenty-four hours in advance. It is like you are trying to win a game long before the whistle blows to start it. There is so much time spent worrying and fretting that in the process we lose the opportunity for deep restorative sleep, in exchange for nothing but more worries, fear, and stress.

The mind at its foundation is a problem solver, and this is the reason we humans have been able to survive for as long as we have. In the past, we had to develop a language so we could communicate to each other what we wanted, needed, and felt. We had to figure out currency systems to exchange goods; thus we have pieces of paper we call "money." And one of our greatest feats, one we are continuing to develop, is learning how to get along with each other and build well-functioning societies.

One of the basic reasons your mind keeps churning at night is simply because it is continuously trying to find some meaning in the chaos of information you are still mulling over from the day's many complex experiences. This is both mental and physical. The untrained mind has the overzealous expectation of finding peace and simplicity among the confusion and disorder of the restless mind. Therefore, you get exhausted from turning the same questions over and over again in your mind.

Below are examples of these kinds of detrimental thought patterns that should be let go from your mental processing.

• *Rehashing the history of things you have done or things others have done to you, making yourself a victim.* It is a waste of time to try to figure out why people did or did not do the things of the past. You cannot change the past, you cannot make things happen differently, you can never truly know what is in another's mind, and you certainly should not continuously beat yourself up. All these points only act to create more discord in the mind by complicating it with emotions such as guilt and fear. Yes, we all do things we wish we didn't. And we will always wonder if things would have come out differently if we had studied or played harder. But what's done is done, and while the past makes fascinating chatter, it does nothing in the way of finding solutions to cure anger, nervousness, or depression. You will never find simplified answers in this pile of chaotic data of the mind, so seeking them in this manner only acts to further complicate the issues at hand.

• *Future fears are another pile of useless data.* It is a useless task to try to fix things the day before. But people often wake up in the middle of the night trying to decide what they are going to do the next day to fix something. The body gets the message that it is time to start energizing the organs and muscles—not to go to sleep, which is what you really need to do. Bottom line: stop trying to solve problems for the next day while you need to rest and sleep.

• *Rehashing situations that make you angry or upset.* Too many times we replay situations that upset us that happened days or even years before, and to no surprise, we get upset over and over again. There are even situations that may not have happened, but that we imagine are going to happen, that upset us. I remember one man who continued to imagine asking for a raise from his boss, and in this scene he continued to be turned down over and over again. He was upset for a month with this reoccurring thought, and one day he went in and quit. (His boss was actually going to give him a raise, but did not get the opportunity.) Result: loss of sleep, loss of rational thinking, and loss of money.

• *Developing performance anxiety of the sleep itself.* Too often individuals who have trouble with sleep begin to think about this problem as a failure in performing some competitive task. I have heard people say, "I will be facing another failure tonight." So they begin to make two mistakes: they begin to program themselves all day for failure to sleep, and they try too hard to get to sleep. Sleeping is the art of letting go of competition and demand, not the act of self-determination. This kind of thinking defeats the process. Sleep is not a competition or something you fail in. It is not something in which you can make grades or be given a rating. You do not get trophies or ribbons.

Not only does this mode of thinking make the process of finding deep restorative sleep a negative experience, it is totally unnecessary and detrimental to the process.

## *Letting Go of Negative Thoughts*

Begin to put your mind in neutral. This may sound like an easy thing to do, but the right mind-set for sleep is a habit that must be practiced. Like a car's transmission when you are trying to park it and continually putting it into drive, your mind cannot go into sleep cycles when you are still trying to go 100 miles per hour on the freeway. There are two methods that I recommend, and they can work by themselves or in combination.

### Method One: Focus on the Present Process

Begin the process by focusing on the present, eliminating thoughts about the past or future. If you become aware of drifting into these no-no areas, immediately stop that thought pattern and resume present thoughts. Do this in a way that is gentle, like training a puppy. If you begin to put pressure and discontent into these kinds of thoughts, they only grow stronger. So easily and softly get your mind back into the present by focusing on something in the present. A great tool for focusing your attention here is to be mindful of your breathing. Begin to feel how the skin feels with each breath, then how the air feels when it enters your lungs or exits your nose. Place all your attention on your breath and put everything else out of your mind. As other thoughts or sensations grab your attention, softly and gently bring your mind back to the breath. This takes some discipline, and it does absolutely no good to beat yourself up if your mind wanders. Also, it is not necessary to change or try to control your breathing patterns; simply observe them.

**Method Two: Music Travel Distraction**
Focus your attention on something audible. Select some music that you enjoy, or better, music that has no particular melody, such as new age music. I prefer Native American flute or drum music for relaxation, but there are tastes for everyone. Just remember that you do not want inspirational songs, especially those you can sing along with, and you sure don't want depressing songs. Listed below are some recommendations for music selections for your interest.

- *Johannes Linstead, Guitarra del Fuego* (Real Music)
- *Lullaby: A Collection* (Music for Little People)
- *Lumia Nights* (Neuronion Records)
- *Miracles* (healingmusic.com)
- *Spirit Keepers* (New World Music, Inc.)
- *Wind Riders* (Talking Taco Music, Inc.)

Sleep is intended to be joyful as well as restorative, not a demand for performance or an expectation we place on ourselves. You do not have to become a sleep athlete to understand that the winner is always you.

## One More Interesting Method

An extremely simple exercise I encourage you to consider is chewing gum for a few minutes before you go to bed. Yes, it may sound like a basic action, but believe it or not, the research done on chewing gum to relieve stress is pretty impressive. The act of chewing gum pumps healing blood into the frontal lobe, where executive functions are controlled, and into your temporal lobe, where stressful emotions are found. There is clear evidence that stress is reduced by as much as 50 percent by chewing gum, and you may gain some IQ points while you're at it. I recommend chewing gums that are recommended by the American Dental Association to help prevent tooth decay along with your efforts.

Another easy technique you can do is to use a powerful mouth rinse. If you have bacteria working in your gums, it can create bad results for the rest of your body. Anything you eat can be affected by this bacteria, and you don't want any bad guys holding up the train to recovery.

## Concluding Remarks

Scientists were once convinced that the brain ceased growing somewhere between the ages of sixteen and twenty-five. Damaged brain cells were considered dead and never to be resurrected. PTSD was considered one step away from terminal degeneration. We have come a long way since then.

With the latest discoveries about brain plasticity and methods of brain healing, we have lifted the curtain on a whole new plan that offers hope. The hardest step is the first one, but we are lucky that there are many routes to brain healing available, from hyperbaric chamber therapy to nutrition to proper sleep. If PTSD has a basis in an injury to the brain, then it only makes sense to heal the brain first. That way it can function at its best and deal with the psychological challenge it may face for adaptation.

The good news is that the brain has amazing rebounding force to renew itself within its inborn capacities. We know these facts from the amazing accounts of the brain plasticities, in which people have used the resources of the "back-up systems" in the brain to walk and talk again. Individuals with only half the brain volume as normal people have had normal lives without realizing any limitations. With only small encouragement from technology in the medical world, it is reasonable and expected that this recovery can be accomplished successfully.

# Chapter Three

# Step Two: Cleansing the Brain of Toxins and Poisons

Ruth was a soldier in World War II, but she did not develop PTSD from her experiences in the war. Rather, her PTSD was related to a traumatic hospital experience. She had gone in for knee surgery at age sixty-five with the objective of eliminating the pain she experienced while walking. But something went terribly wrong. The surgeon and the medical staff present were all horrified when Ruth began to jerk, waking from the anesthesia just as they were transferring her off the surgery table. Ruth's sudden and unexpected movement caused the staff to lose their grip, and they dropped her to the floor. As she landed, her knee bent back and sideways at a ninety degree angle. In addition to this traumatic injury to her knee, she also suffered a chipped bone in her pelvis and a broken elbow. She was given enough anesthesia to put her back into a deep sleep and was then carted off to the critical care unit.

Like so many PTSD patients, her brain was not directly injured from the traumatic event itself; however, the trauma etched a major stress response in her brain, and it was this stress response that played itself every time she tried to enter the sleep state. The symptoms of PTSD were clear; she couldn't get the deep restorative sleep she needed, and the brief moments she did sleep were filled with constant traumatizing nightmares of the fall. She dreaded nighttime when she knew she would be afraid of letting her guard down and feeling the horrific pain again, but she so badly needed deep, restful sleep.

Her first attempt to deal with this was through sleep medication, which gave her a mixed blessing: she achieved relief from the deep fatigue she was experiencing from lack of sleep, but on the other hand she was still experiencing the horrifying nightmares when she did sleep. Though she had never been much of a social drinker, alcohol soon became her closest and only friend. The alcohol masked the pain and gave her a false sense of security where she felt some control and less anxiety. But it also brought her more and more isolation as well as all the baggage associated with alcohol abuse.

The lapse of control due to the grogginess of drinking then led to her use of marijuana, and from there she eventually found her way into using pain medications. By the time she walked into our office, she had a laundry list of drugs she was taking in an attempt to squash the overbearing burden of her trauma. She was desperate for help.

What we found was that Ruth was not dealing with an addiction, as she had thought when she first came in. This was because she was not so much trying to get high as much as she was seeking to escape the traumatic experience itself. But she was definitely presenting toxic brain patterns that needed to be repaired.

Thus, we needed to repair the damaged areas of her brain while also detoxifying and healing the inflamed brain. This needed to happen before we could make any headway on the other underlying issues within her PTSD diagnosis.

We ran tests to discover her levels of toxicity and exposure to pesticides and heavy metals. Just as we had predicted, she was showing extremely high toxicity levels in the brain (which is actually more common than you may think, as will be discussed later). Though the toxicities from the alcohol and drugs she had been taking were evident, there were also surprisingly high levels of mercury and lead in her system. Because of the high environmental exposures to these heavy metals in the area where she lived, we felt that there may have been a predisposition to the joint pains she had that led to the surgery.

Our goal was to detoxify the brain and to stop the

poisonous reactions of the elements that were interfering with the process of healing. Once we did, Ruth's brain healed quickly as we observed her cognitive functions return rapidly, though she still complained of lack of sleep and torturous nightmares.

Now that she was neurologically healthy enough to process information, we could begin to gain control of her emotions. At this stage she went through the systematic desensitization program addressed in this chapter and removed the fears associated with the surgical accident. She slept thirteen hours that night, and we encouraged her to take advantage of the opportunity to let her brain rest in order to heal to the maximum capacity.

Until Ruth's decline into the PTSD turmoil of alcohol and medication abuse, she had kept a very stable community of friends, and her family lived nearby. This support system was very helpful in making the rest of her journey a breeze. When we saw her last at the clinic, she reported a new strength and a brand-new mission in life with an air of confidence.

While Ruth's recovery may be remarkable, the damage she suffered is, unfortunately, quite common among those with PTSD. In the previous step we discussed healing the brain damage and how important that is to enabling the brain to face the next steps of PTSD recovery. Similarly, the brain cannot function at its best if it is hampered by toxins and poisons. And as we will see, the toxins quite often find their way into the brain, due to reasons both intentional and unintentional. To truly continue on the road to recovery then, the next step is to detoxify the brain of these toxic substances.

## How Does the Toxic Brain Damage Happen?

The brain is undoubtedly our most reactive organ, responding to every function in the body. This includes the sensitivity of your skin, movement of your body from one place to another, and reactions to stimuli such as pain, body temperature, outside temperature, and the million and one functions all occurring simultaneously within your body. So almost everything we do or experience affects the brain in some way. And therefore often, through the things we do or the environments we find ourselves in, we unknowingly mistreat our brain instead of nurturing and protecting it the way we should. Those who suffer from PTSD are even more prone to toxic damage, because they are trying different ways to cure or live with their condition. But this is like trying to figure out why an automobile engine is running rough while at the same time putting water in the gas tank. The driver might be trying as hard as he can, but the engine simply is not getting the right mixture of fuel and will never work properly until it is "detoxified," so to speak.

The most common toxins that PTSD victims are exposed to while trying to deal with their condition are alcohol and drugs. Like Ruth, when we put substances such as these into our bodies, they affect the brain in ways we do not intend and can produce very puzzling and frustrating outcomes. You can imagine then the confusion that results when victims of PTSD mess around with unnatural drugs and substances that are already known to cause major changes in the brain, and add these effects on top of the damage already sustained by their brain.

But the toxins our brains are exposed to don't always come from things we intentionally put in our bodies. You never know where you might be intoxicating or possibly damaging your brain with outside substances.

Here is a striking example of a situation when extreme brain toxicity and/or damage can occur from something you never would have thought possible. Have you or someone you know ever lived in a brand-new home? You may not be aware that new homes can have high amounts of formaldehyde in the walls and carpeting, as these are added to shut down organic aging and restrict cellular processing of the products in homes. However, there is the danger that your exposure to this substance may also consequently shut down your own brain's cellular processing. This scenario is more common that you think. I have witnessed cases in which people have become paralyzed physically and immobilized psychologically to the edge of life or death due to this type of exposure.

Parasites found in your intestines can also create adverse reactions to your brain chemistry. The majority of the neurotransmitters that are the main interaction agents in your brain are born in the intestines, and thus these parasites can cause damage later affecting your brain.

So all you need to do is avoid these toxins, right? Unfortunately it's not as easy as that. The problem is that very few people have the proper understanding to know what needs to change in their behavior, diet, and thinking in order to find happiness, much less change their brain chemistry. We live in a society that advocates medication as the solution for our daily problems. Many people line up for antianxiety medications because they can't handle the stresses in their lives. And many doctors prescribe all these drugs, numbing the patient's brain just when the opportunities to find true healing are emerging.

This is not to say that medication is evil or not given in the best interest of a person, but it is certainly not the cure. And we have to face the facts: there are no medications available to cure PTSD. Further, medications, pesticides, chemicals, and drugs are not only ineffective, they also leave behind a toxic aftermath in the PTSD brain and body that must be repaired. The body has to then attempt as best it can to dispose of these foreign chemicals, often leaving it to the overworked kidneys to cleanse the system. (Anyone who has lived through a hangover from one night's indulgence can vouch for the damage toxins can do in just twenty-four hours.) For the PTSD brain to truly heal, it must be cleansed of its toxins so that it can function at its best level. Fortunately, there are many good methods available for detoxifying the brain.

## Is Your Brain Contaminated?

Following the process of the Compass RESET Program, you must first determine if your brain is suffering due to toxicity. The probability is quite high that your brain has some level of toxicity interfering with its executive functioning, no matter your lifestyle or where you live. This is because the environment we live in is simply so precarious to human welfare. Even natives in the remote jungles of South America and Africa have to deal with vicious parasites and dangerous health practices. So you can imagine the number of toxins a person in an urban or developed region is exposed to on a regular basis.

Consider the tables below that show the direct impact on brain function, documented in studies, from the exposure to heavy metals. Note that there are overlaps of these conditions, and many interact with other biological organic functions to create other seriously damaging side effects. For example, exposure to lead often interacts with the thyroid gland, and low energy, depression, and low cognitive functioning can result from that one condition alone.

## Effects of Exposure to Heavy Metals on Cognitive Abilities

| | |
|---|---|
| Cadmium (common from manufacturing waste) | Motor dysfunction |
| | Decreased IQ |
| | Hyperactivity |
| | Hypoactivity |
| Lead | Learning difficulties |
| | Decreased IQ |
| | Impulsivity |
| | Attention deficit |
| | Hyperactivity |
| | Violence |
| Manganese | Brain damage |
| | Motor dysfunction |
| | Attention deficit |
| | Compulsive disorder |
| Mercury | Visual Impairment |
| | Learning disabilities |
| | Attention deficit |
| | Motor dysfunction |
| | Memory impairment |

## Effects of Exposure to Solvents on Cognitive Abilities

| | |
|---|---|
| Ethanol (alcohol) | Learning difficulties |
| | Attention deficit |
| | Memory impairment |
| | Eating/sleeping disorders |
| | Mental retardation |
| Styrene | Hypoactivity |
| | Lack of inhibition |
| Toluene | Learning disabilities |
| | Speech deficits |
| | Motor dysfunction |
| Trichloroethylene | Hyperactivity |
| | Lack of inhibition |
| Xylene | Motor dysfunction |
| | Learning difficulties |
| | Memory impairment |

## Effects of Exposure to Pesticides on Cognitive Abilities

| | |
|---|---|
| Organochlorines/DDT | Hyperactivity |
| | Decreased energy/effort |
| | Decreased coordination |
| | Memory impairment |
| Organophosphates (including DFP, chlorpyrifos, Dursban, dizainon) | Hyperactivity |
| | Attention disorders |

|  | Decreased ability to follow instructions |
|  | Hyperactivity |
|  | Attention problems |

## Effects of Exposure to Other Common Substances on Cognitive Behavior

| PCBs | Learning disabilities |
|  | Attention deficits |
|  | Hyperactivity |
|  | Memory impairments |
| Fluoride | Hyperactivity |
|  | Decreased IQ |

The Environmental Working Group, using data from the USDA and FDA pesticide research bank from 1992 to 1997, has compiled the most contaminated fruits available directly to consumers. It is critical and mandatory that all your fruits and vegetables be washed or even peeled to reduce exposure, as a practical guide.

- Apples
- Celery
- Grapes (from Chile)
- Green beans
- Peaches

- Pears
- Potatoes
- Red raspberries
- Spinach
- Strawberries

The only way to know for sure if your brain has been exposed to toxins is to have some lab tests completed by a physician, but considering how common such exposure is, it is safe to say that your brain could benefit from one of the number of ways available to cleanse it of toxins. Let's take a look at some of the most effective methods for doing so.

## Natural Approaches to Cleansing the Brain

Some of the best ways to cleanse the body of toxins come in natural forms. These natural ingredients have been found to help the cleansing process:

- Alfalfa
- Aloe vera
- Fennel seed
- Flax seed
- Ginger tea
- Grapefruit pectin
- Guar gum
- Licorice root
- Marshmallow root
- Papaya fruit
- Peppermint
- Rhubarb root
- Slippery elm bark

There are several ancient methods of cleansing the body that also work well. These are especially effective for water-soluble elements and aid the body in eliminating toxins through sweating, urinating, and other natural processes. Below is a list of methods that many people have found effective:

- Hot saunas, especially with sesame or juniper oils
- Physical exercise
- Massages, especially for those massage specialists who know how to help the lymph glands release their reserves
- Lemon water
- Very high-fiber diets
- Coffee enemas

There are a wide variety of methods available, and a number of ways to use the different natural ingredients to cleanse your brain and body. Some work better for some than others, so I do not know exactly which will work best for you individually. You should try a number of them until you discover which options are giving you the best results. You should also consult with your doctor on which methods he or she recommends, and he or she can help track your progress.

Here are some of the methods, though, that have produced strong results for many people, and thus are definitely worth exploring.

## *Stimulating the Body's Natural Cleansing Enzymes*

There is general consensus that one of the best ways to nurture the brain is with antioxidants. The chief vitamin antioxidants are vitamins C, E, $B_6$, and $B_{12}$. Mineral antioxidants include selenium, zinc, calcium, and magnesium. Direct supplements can be used to develop an antioxidant army. Here are general guidelines for daily dosages. Please note that they vary according to age, weight, and individual needs. Consult with a specialist to determine your specific needs.

| | |
|---|---|
| Vitamin C | 1,000 mg daily |
| Vitamin E | 400 IU daily |
| Vitamin $B_6$ | 50 mg daily |
| Vitamin $B_{12}$ | 50 mcg daily |
| Calcium | 260 mg daily |
| Magnesium | 160 mg daily |

Supplements are created by synthesizing ingredients of a natural food or substance, which makes it more difficult for the body to recognize and metabolize. However, when these ingredients are consumed within the foods themselves, the correct formula for digestion is natural and has the advantage of better processing. Real food is still the best way to get nutrients. The following foods are major suppliers of antioxidants:

- Asparagus
- Beans
- Beets
- Berries, especially blue-berries and raspberries
- Broccoli
- Brussels sprouts
- Cabbage
- Carrots
- Citrus fruits
- Nuts
- Onions
- Prunes
- Spinach
- Red grapes
- Red peppers
- Sweet potatoes
- Tomatoes
- Watermelon
- Wheat germ

Here are some additional substances that aid in the detoxification process (follow the recommended dosages on the labels):

- **Milk thistle**—used as a liver protectant.

- **Calcium D-glucarate**—allows for increased net elimination of toxins and steroid hormones.

- **N-acetyl-L-cysteine (NAC)**—produces a dramatic acceleration of urinary methylmercury excretion, and has been shown to reduce liver damage.

- **Alpha-ketoglutaric acid (AKA)**—helps detoxify ammonia, very effective as an antioxidative agent.

- **Methylsulfonylmethane (MSM)**—a naturally occurring sulfur compound used in detoxification processes.

- **Taurine**—appears to inhibit catecholamine oxidation in the brain; also required for the formation of bile salts, an important mode of toxin elimination.

- **Methionine**—assists in the removal process for heavy metals as well as aiding in the excretion through the urine.

- **Choline**—acts as a neurotransmitter as well as metabolic enhancer; very important at the cellular level of detoxification; individuals who consume a choline-deficit diet often develop hepatic disease.

- **Betaine anhydrous**—also known as trimethylglycine, a major metabolite of choline; usually found in small amounts in beets, spinach, and seafood.

- **Selenium**—required for the synthesis of a vital antioxidant enzyme that helps detoxify hydrogen peroxide reproduced within cells.

## Colon Cleansing

If you want to get really concerned about how your colon is dealing with your environment, consider that every living thing has at least one parasite that lives within it. It might scare you to see the awful-looking creatures that live within a person's body. And as you learned earlier, such parasites can cause damage that affects brain function.

It might be worth a doctor's visit for a stool sample to rule out the problems of digestive failures and inflammatory reactions of such visitors. Some people even go through a colon cleansing as a routine process and give terrific testimonies about how their lives have changed as a result. If you are interested in doing this, go online and search for "natural detox of the colon" (or liver), and you will find hundreds of such testimonies and products that foster such beliefs.

## Special Natural Supplements for PTSD

The direct influence of nutrition on both the structure and the function of the human brain is being rapidly investigated by researchers and clinical communities. Over the last ten years, a framework has emerged that provides a scientific basis for nutritional supplements and their critical importance. Most importantly, much of the ancient wisdom and clinical intuition is being substantiated, so that those individuals who suffer repressions of intellectual power can prosper with special nutrients and botanicals.

The following list contains a small set of supplements that have been documented as benefiting individuals with neurological problems related to toxicity and can be considered as healing substances. They certainly appear to have powerful impact, although it is strongly suggested that you have a treatment plan and information from a professional in order to have the most immediate impact. (Use the published dosages on the labels as guides.)

- Acetyl-L-carnitine has been used for improvement of several neurological problems, including difficulties with memory, concentration, and mood. This substance occurs naturally in the body as an enhancer of cellular energy by acting as a shuttle between the cytoplasm and the mitochondria for fatty acids. It may also accelerate choline activity, facilitating serotonin pathways and enhancing synaptic transmission.

- Carnosine is a natural substance that has been used to foster frontal lobe function (increased attention and focus) and has a brain-protective function as well. Individuals have been shown to improve in vocabulary and organization, which would show promise for other people with neurological issues in these areas. Interestingly, literature suggests that this substance also possesses neurotransmission activity that modulates enzymatic activities, such as chelating heavy metals.

• The combination of American ginseng (200 mg) and ginkgo biloba (50 mg) has been shown to have significant benefits for individuals with hyperactive-impulsive behaviors or high anxiety—both traits related to the social problems associated with PTSD. There has also been improvement in the performances of quality of memory at the highest dose and speed of attention at a mid-dose range.

• Ginkgo biloba in daily doses of 120 to 240 mg can improve symptoms of memory loss, depression, and tinnitus (ringing in the ears), especially if the symptoms are related to trauma. It serves as a free-radical scavenger (which is a major aid in the prevention of disease) but may have direct effects on the cholinergic system. This may explain its positive impact on acute and chronic cognitive-enhancing effects related to PTSD.

• American ginseng has been shown to enhance central nervous system activity (brain and spinal cord), decrease fatigue, and increase motor activity. Ginseng has antide-pressant, antipsychotic, anticonvulsant, analgesic, anti-pyretic, and ulcer-protective qualities. Psychologically it has been shown to inhibit conditioned avoidance responses. Interestingly related to toxicity, it has an anti-inflammatory quality and increases gastrointestinal action, thereby decreasing constipation. In combina-tion with Panax ginseng, attention problems and symp-toms of attention-deficit disorder were greatly reduced. Panax ginseng has been shown to have beneficial effects on the immune cells of individuals with chronic fatigue syndrome, a syndrome associated with individuals with PTSD, attention-deficit disorder, or autism.

## Contaminated in the Line of Duty

So far we have discussed common contaminants that are dangerous to all of us. But for the veteran who has experi-enced the many toxic elements in war, including the hot lead from explosives and ammunition, the toxicity they face will be far more intense.

One example of this comes to mind for me whenever I think of our soldiers and toxins. George was a walking miracle after he completed his second round of duty. But he was also a walking time bomb in terms of his PTSD, and his rage had become uncontrollable. The symptoms he experienced while on military duty were quite shocking. He reported the shades of his urine changing day to day, as well as some astonishing colors found in his stools. To say the least, he was not happy, and each day was a struggle to keep his anger from destroying his opportunities. He had allergies to everything, which created severe itching in his genital area. On top of all of this was an extreme body odor that smelled strongly acidic and repelled the bravest of our staff. Even the kindest therapist had to direct a fourteen-inch fan in his direction just so they could have a conversation.

In spite of these conditions, George understood that we were determined to work the system with the ultimate goal of healing. His belief in us kept the process going.

The results were outstanding. Over a period of just six weeks we could see (and smell) the difference. George felt better, and most of his symptoms were decreasing. I could imagine his brain had been just as inflamed and reactive as his skin.

George's case shows that our soldiers are exposed to the most extreme forms of toxins in the line of duty. The weaponry of today's soldiers has advanced far beyond the guns and dynamite of our country's earliest wars. Many of the present-day arsenals are top secret, making the job of treating soldiers difficult because we have no idea what chemicals and/or heavy metals they are exposed to. We do know there are uranium bullets that can pierce the side of a battleship and all sorts of explosive chemicals that make up specific high-tech rifles. Not only can the high-level noises of these weapons injure the brain, but so can exposure to the toxic chemicals when handling the ammunition. When these concoctions explode and the intense heat creates a deadly gas, the result is major toxicity of the brain and possible brain damage.

Besides weapons and chemicals, there are also increasingly more environmental issues, usually involving the toxic contaminated dust. One of the most commonly known toxins is Agent Orange from the Vietnam struggle and the soldiers' problems that resulted from that substance. There are also the toxins soldiers are exposed to from the enemy's actions. Remember that deadly chemicals and gasses have been used to kill people in most wars at one time or another, and even deadly viruses have been released in an attempt to injure soldiers. War is not pretty from any angle, and the most vulnerable organ in the body is the brain.

## The Deep Cleanse

Thankfully it is possible to dig out the toxic elements of war by "cleansing" the brain. This is accomplished through the use of substances that bind to any heavy metal molecules in the body so they will be extracted from your system.

Modifilan, a brown seaweed extract, is one of the most effective of these substances. It was used to help treat victims of the Chernobyl disaster who were suffering from radiation poisoning and is readily available today over the counter. It contains the following beneficial ingredients (as reported on www.modifilan-seaweedextract.com):

- **Alginate:** this is a natural absorbent of radioactive elements, heavy metals, and free radicals. It has the unique ability of binding heavy metals and radioactive elements to its own molecules. As the alginate cannot be broken down by bile or saliva and cannot be absorbed by the body, it is secreted from the body together with the heavy metals and radioactive substances.

- **Organic Iodine:** The thyroid gland, which controls metabolism and promotes maturation of the nervous system, needs iodine as fuel. Iodine is important for thyroid disorders, whether under- or overactive.

- **Fucoxanthin:** this is found in brown seaweed and promotes abdominal weight loss as well as helps to fight diabetes.

- **Fucoidan:** this causes certain types of rapidly growing cancer cells to self-destruct. Promoting apoptosis (self-destruction of cancer cells), fucoidan helps to naturally eliminate harmful cells from organism.

• **Laminarin:** this is a polysaccharide helpful in the prevention and treatment of cardiovascular diseases.

## *Oral Chelation*

Another form of deep cleanse is oral chelation. Chelex-100 is an effective medication used at clinics to cleanse the body of certain toxins. It contains substances that bond with toxic elements and heavy metals to form big enough molecules for the filtering system of the body to put them into the urine system. It also includes vitamin C and glutathione so that the substances don't just go from one organ to another without leaving the body.

The use of Chelex-100 is a very sensitive process that doctors and clinicians monitor closely. My clinic has been doing this process for over five years, and only two people have noted problems. Both of these individuals said they did not feel well, so the process was stopped immediately. I mention Chelex-100 as a possible method for a medical approach, but it requires medical supervision and its availability can be limited. I would certainly recommend a very clear understanding of the process with a reputable physician if interested.

# Picking and Choosing

This chapter has mentioned a wide array of products available to you as a way of decontaminating the toxic PTSD brain and discovering the paths to making positive changes. It is not my intent to recommend all of them at once, because some will work better than others for certain individuals. You can pick and choose the ones you have the most faith in that give you the best results.

Decontamination doesn't happen overnight, and sometimes things seem to change in bizarre ways. This can be very disconcerting if you didn't know about or expect it.

Choosing these products and procedures is also a lifestyle adjustment. As I shared in Ruth's story, too many PTSD victims make poor choices in their search for change. They are not bad or morally challenged people, but they are often desperate and afraid. Finding answers via alcohol and drugs will not work, although these may be the only options they knew about. And you now know better. And when you know better, you do better.

Detoxifying your brain is a key step in your recovery, but you can't expect to know how to do it on your own. This is why the critical decision to reach out and accept guidance is so important. This is the time and place when family and community can help, even though there can be resistance. This is when faith in another human being can truly mean the most, because the next step involves resetting your mind so you can better live and love those closest to you in life. It is a step that is difficult but one that if done right will begin to reopen all the best things in your life to you.

# CHAPTER FOUR

# Step Three: Making Reconnections and Taking Control of the Disoriented Brain

Rosa left her family of two young children to fulfill her duty in Iraq, only to come back as a stranger to them. It was as if she no longer had the maternal instincts she once had. As she explained, "I felt I had been traumatized into not knowing how to do things I had done before routinely. And it was not lack of remembering, it was not having the natural instincts and feelings anymore. I felt like they had died back there."

While she previously enjoyed being with her family, she now wanted to escape. She felt clumsy and like she was role-playing the act of caring to make her family and friends comfortable. This sense of faking would lead her to depression and loss of connection to those she loved. Before her tour of duty in Iraq, she hadn't been a verbally expressive individual, but now she had to fight to restrain herself from blurting out hostile words. Rosa was most uncomfortable in church, where she felt like a phony when parishioners asked about her faith, which she had openly expressed before, but now had no passion or any feelings for at all. She was dead emotionally.

Rosa recalls this stage as the hell of her lifetime, and you can understand how difficult this must be. To experience the total alteration of her personality, from being a genuine and sincerely caring person to being totally aloof and even paranoid of her own family, was extremely traumatic. She had lost herself and didn't care.

# The Disoriented Brain

Once you have healed the physical damage to your brain, the next step in recovery is to restore the connections in your brain that allow you to function in normal life. I refer to this phase as the "broken arm" stage of PTSD. If you have ever broken your arm (or any part of your body that moves), you know that when the cast is taken off it hurts to bend it. It is like you have to learn to use it all over again. This is because while you aren't using your arm, the nerves in your muscles detach from the bundle that controls your arm and hook up with a bundle that is more active. Your other arm might get stronger because it is more active and gets more attention from the brain. But once the cast is off, your body has to learn to use the other arm again.

The same is true for your brain. Rosa's brain, like that of

many PTSD sufferers, has programmed itself to make itself more resistant to harm at the sake of losing normal function. But once back in the normal world, the brain needs to return to normal functioning.

This process is not always automatic, though, even after you have healed the brain of any physical damage or toxins. An airman does not simply get into the cockpit of an F-22 aircraft and take off just because he desires to be a pilot. He has to go through training. Someone has to show him how to be a pilot. Similarly, you cannot assume that if you have a healthy brain, it will know how to operate at full throttle. You have to go through a lot of brain training to reach that level of efficiency. And that is where Rosa needed to start— she had to reteach her brain to operate again.

## The Upside and Downside of Brain Plasticity

The problem of brain reconnections is both caused and cured by an incredible thing known as brain plasticity. Brain plasticity means that your brain is always changing and reacting to the demands placed on it. There are "circuits" in your brain composed of neurons that serve as connectors, like little electrical cords running everywhere, except that they are living cells and not machines.

How do they work? Think about the latest in computer

printers. There are now very affordable wireless printers so that everyone in your household can print documents from their laptops without being hard-wired to the printer. The two pieces of equipment have an electronic handshake that is sent to connect each other; they are like two neurons talking to each other. The "magic" of the wireless communication helps them talk to each other and send a document to be printed. If for some reason there is a disruption in the communication that is taking place, the document will print incorrectly or not at all.

One of the principles of brain plasticity is that these neurons hook up according to what is available, which is likely what the body needs. For example, if your finger is cut off, all the neurons that were connected to that finger would not die but switch to another operation, usually a finger next to it. It makes the other finger better, perhaps compensating for the lost one. This is likely one of the reasons why people who are blind report improvements in their hearing or sense of touch.

When Rosa was placed in a situation of survival, all of her neurons hooked onto survival mechanisms and left behind her traditional hookups, like taking care of her children and home and socializing with friends and family. With the fear of combat producing full-throttle adrenal juices pumping in her veins and arteries, and without a need to focus on her relationships at home, she would be directing as many of her neurons as possible toward not getting killed. She would also try to shut down her emotional switchboard to avoid going crazy or being paralyzed by fear from the memories of her experiences. Her memory switchboard would be pulling plugs as fast as it could to forget what she saw or heard.

In just a matter of weeks, the concussive sounds and contaminated environment of war deprogrammed Rosa's brain in a drastic way. When she returned home after her deployment, she was still disoriented and very afraid. It's no wonder so many PTSD soldiers want to go back to the war where their brains don't suffer from the anxieties that greet them once home. To them, the war is easier to face than coming home and recognizing that you are not feeling the compassion and parental instincts you felt before you left.

Fortunately, there is a better solution than going back to war, or reexperiencing the pain or trauma of the event that caused your PTSD. By using the methods in this chapter, you can learn to reset the connections in your brain back to those of normal life so you can once again live and feel as you did before the events that caused your PTSD. Let's take a look at how to put this in action.

## Do You Have a Disoriented Brain?

This phase is where the strategic and empowering aspects of the Compass RESET are so critical. The first steps to determine if you indeed have areas within your brain that need to be reoriented. To do this, I have identified several thinking patterns that impair brain processing, and developed a questionnaire to help you identify if you are having a problem in those areas. This test allows you to become aware of the possibility that your brain may not be operating at its full potential.

Note how the following statements pertain to you by marking always true (AT), sometimes true (ST), rarely true (RT), or never true (NT).

1. *I feel that I am a misfit in my community and family.*
   AT  ST  RT  NT

2. *I feel numb to my emotions.*
   AT  ST  RT  NT

3. *I just can't stop my mind from entering a flood of rage toward others, even for little things.*
   AT  ST  RT  NT

4. *I get very obsessive about wanting things done my way.*
   AT  ST  RT  NT

5. *I can't sleep because my mind keeps ruminating about something.*
   AT  ST  RT  NT

6.  *I want to be alone and away from everybody.*
    AT   ST   RT   NT

7.  *No one really understands me; I don't understand myself.*
    AT   ST   RT   NT

8.  *I am easily distracted by other events.*
    AT   ST   RT   NT

9.  *I have trouble listening or even caring about what another person is saying to me.*
    AT   ST   RT   NT

10. *I have nightmares.*
    AT   ST   RT   NT

11. *I have fears about irrational things, such as closed or open places and people.*
    AT   ST   RT   NT

12. *I am angry and can't shake the emotion.*
    AT   ST   RT   NT

Scoring: Assign a score of 3 to every AT you circled, a 2 to every ST, and a 1 for every RT, and total all of the twelve items for a score within the range of 0–36. Compare your scores to the following ranges:

24–36    Your brain is disoriented to the point that you do not trust yourself.

18–23    Your brain is disoriented for some problems in your life.

11–17    There are some areas in which you get confused.

0–10     Your brain appears to be oriented to the point that you are not being confused.

If you scored 11 or higher, the following techniques are designed to get you back on track. I can be very positive that this phase will be successful for you, but it does require commitment.

## The Basic Exercise of Life: Breathing

In my forty years as a psychologist, I have seen individuals with PTSD breathe in only two ways, both of them wrong and both of them endangering their brains for further problems. The most common pattern is what I call the "rabbit rate," because you can also observe this pattern in rabbits when they are being hunted. The pattern consists of short, shallow breaths at a rate around twenty to thirty breaths per minute. Sometimes these breaths are so quick that they can't be measured at all because you can't see any movement in the chest. This pattern is consistent with chronic anxiety. It is as if they don't want to make a sound with their breathing in fear of getting caught.

When you take more than fifteen breaths per minute, you signal to the rest of your body, especially the brain, that you are stressing out. This pattern triggers the fight-or-flight response in your entire body, especially the brain, which has kept humankind in the game since the caveman days. To experience this for yourself, try this experiment: Purposely breathe in and out at a rate of twenty air exchanges per minute. After two minutes of this, if someone hasn't called the guys in white coats, you'll note that you feel agitated. That's because you've triggered some very primal instincts.

The natural response when you are in a panic is to seek out a cause for that panic. Sometimes we attribute the panic to the wrong causes or memories. And if you have a recent memory album full of fears, it is easy to understand why you might get seriously concerned if your memory keeps going back to bullets coming at you and trying to know where to run to avoid bombs that have been planted.

The second most common pattern is hyperventilation (which may be the end result of having rabbit breath). Most of us have seen this when someone can't catch his or her breath. They are in panic mode and often fear death. This is certainly not the time to scare them into that thought by dragging them off to the hospital.

Both of these patterns are detrimental to the brain because they disrupt the oxygen intake most needed for use in thinking and memory. The short breath pattern acts only to produce the minimum amount of air required, and hyperventilation is too much and therefore imbalances the interchange of $O_2$ and $CO_2$. The brain becomes starved for air, which puts it on the verge of risky decision making and fear responses.

Take the stressful situation of taking a test as an example. Some of the behaviors you can recognize as signs of disorientation of the brain include:

- You hold your breath like you are pushing the answers to your brain.

- When you can't remember something you think you should know, you get frustrated and strain the brain to remember.

- Your vision gets blurry.

- You start yawning or hiccupping.

• You have trouble stopping your thinking on one topic or subject in order to shift to another problem.

• You can't be creative when under pressure; you can only come up with poor solutions.

• You make a lot of simple errors.

• You begin to think of a hundred different things rather than focusing on the questions and answers at hand.

• Sometimes you can't take the test seriously and begin to only think of humorous and cynical responses to the questions.

If you find yourself experiencing any of these breathing patterns, learning to adjust them can help you not only solve your breathing issues, but also build reconnections in your brain that will help you function normally in everyday life. So let's take a look at a number of strategies designed to help you correct your breathing patterns.

## Breathing Strategies

Breathing is as easy as, well, breathing, once you learn to pay attention to doing it in the proper way. It's the epitome of natural healing. Here are techniques for learning to control your breathing patterns to improve your health and performance.

**Full Breath**

This pattern can be helpful when you are very anxious and need to gain some emotional control. When you are feeling angry or stressed, breathing in this pattern helps you regain your sense of composure. This is also an extremely helpful pattern for controlling anxiety when you are trying to make big decisions.

The three areas of most importance to concentrate on are the chest, stomach, and shoulders. You will not be able to control all three from the start, but given practice and time, you will be able to advance to each area.

For the first step, place your lower hand on the navel and the other on the chest. Begin by breathing into your lower hand in your stomach area while keeping the chest stable.

Once you have enough practice with that technique and are convinced you have a general understanding of that region of movement, start breathing in a way so that only the chest area is moving and the stomach area remains stable. This can be very tricky for some individuals and may require some coaching from stress-management experts.

After those experiences are clear, breathe only through the shoulders by slightly raising them up with each breath in, while keeping both the chest and stomach stable. After all three levels are done, begin to breathe by moving all three areas (chest, stomach, and shoulders). It takes a little practice, but most people report a sense of relaxation very quickly as they open up these capacities. Try breathing into your stomach area and following the wave of movement as it goes into the chest, then the shoulders, and then exhaling back down, noticing the wavelike motion.

This method is fun to watch on the brain monitor because it shows a beautiful blend of frequencies. It's like a symphony in which all the instruments blend together in perfect harmony. And, staying with that metaphor, this method actually helps you get into harmony with yourself. When you experience stress and tension, it is often because you are not centered or emotionally stable. Little things may be bothering you and knocking you off balance. When you feel out of synch and edgy, use this technique to get yourself back on track.

Think of a very stressful situation, such as a memory of giving a speech to a large group of people. Rate how stressful this situation was to you with a ranking from one (low impact) to ten (highest impact). While you are imagining this situation, assume this breathing pattern for five minutes. After the five minutes have passed, if you are still thinking of it, rate how stressful it is to you now, using the same one to ten scale. This can be a very important method of letting go of stress and burdens when you need to be strong in order to meet a challenge.

This full-breath breathing pattern is extremely popular, especially among people who have trouble sleeping. Billy, like probably half of the people in this country, had difficulty sleeping, a central factor in PTSD diagnosis. He'd be lucky to get in three hours of true rest a night. However, Billy was able to learn and apply techniques for creating a restful pattern of sleep. Once he'd mastered the technique, he began to sleep restfully and make better choices in times when he became anxious.

## Alternate Nostrils

The next method might seem a bit unusual at first. It's okay to have fun with this one but, as strange as it sounds, it is actually rooted in ancient East Indian practices. It is a method for breaking thought patterns when you are stuck or can't seem to escape self-defeating behaviors. Maybe you can't stop thinking about someone who hurt your feelings. Or maybe you have been obsessing over an event or memory. This is a way to break free of that pattern so you can focus your mind on more constructive thinking.

The method is to consciously breathe through alternate nostrils. (It is okay to use your fingers on the outside of your nostrils to accomplish this process.) Breathe in one nostril by closing off the other, and when you've done a cycle of exhalation and inhalation, close that nostril and breathe through a complete cycle through the other. Repeat the alternating pattern several times in a relaxed manner.

You'll notice something very interesting happening to your brain. It lights up on the brain monitor, one section after the other. First, it might be your temporal lobes, then your frontal, then toward the back of the brain, or in some varying progression. It is like watching a neon message board flickering on at various times. It may seem chaotic, but out of chaos comes calm. Your brain is doing a reshuffle. It is clearing connections so that you can find a fresh solution.

You can experiment with this technique by focusing on a problem or concern that has been nagging you, like a song playing over and over in your mind. Remember that your goal is to get unstuck from the nagging thought or problem. You will feel some confusion after two or three minutes and you might want to stop, but don't. Keep breathing in this pattern until you can no longer think about the problem. You are cleansing your mind.

This technique worked well for Rosa, who had a lot of worries nagging her. She was lost and all she could think about every waking hour were her anxieties and fears—and since she couldn't sleep, that meant twenty-four hours a day. After practicing this technique for a period of time, Rosa found much relief from these nagging tendencies of her mind.

*Overview of Breathing*

Breathing techniques have been used to assist control of the mind for hundreds of years. They can be very powerful tools, yet we often dismiss them too easily. Breath control is a time-proven method for controlling anxiety and unreasonable fears. It's also much cheaper than prescription drugs. After all, the air is free.

## Body Movements and Brain Function

Another method of reconnecting your brain and taking control is through exercise. Research has shown that exercise can be just as therapeutic as psychotherapy. There are many good reasons why these results are true, including the improved breathing that comes from exerting effort every day, as discussed in the previous section. When you exercise, you breathe more deeply and allow your body and brain to coordinate their healing mechanisms.

We have been practicing physical movement as a medical cure for as long as we have recorded history. Native Americans danced around campfires when trying to solve tribal problems. For centuries, the Irish people cured depression by swimming long distances around Ireland. The Japanese have traditionally performed tai chi exercises to ease and focus the mind. Yoga has an amazing systematic process in which specific mental processes are tied to precise movements. Stresses related to memories that need to be released are a focus of spine alignment, and unless you can release these pent-up emotions, it is difficult, even painful, to accomplish a pose.

Physical exercise has the added benefit of stimulating the body's internal chemistry. It is like you have your own drugstore inside, and each substance is bought by effort. The movement of the joints stimulates the release of endorphin neurotransmitters, which are the basis for feeling joy and happiness as well as the reduction of pain. That boosts the production of serotonin, which reduces depression and anxiety. An overabundance of these transmitters can create an intense psychological high. Several studies have noted that exercise can be more effective for depression than medication. Working out simply beats popping pills.

But you should be cautious about overdoing it. You don't want to burn out your body or your brain by pushing yourself too hard. Excessive exercise can cause inflammation that sends toxins into the brain. When you push your body beyond its capacities, it produces cortisol, a hormone that stresses the brain. Problems with memory and concentration can result. So, get off the couch for the good of your body and your brain, but don't run yourself, or them, into the ground. Consider the effective exercise methods on the following pages.

## Individual Exercise Methods

Many parts of your brain are affected positively when you perform individual exercises, like dancing or swimming. There is ample evidence that exercises requiring balance and coordination can ease the symptoms of PTSD, providing better mental focus.

The areas of the motor ridge (in the center of your brain) and the frontal lobe coordinate thoughts and executive functions. A gentle workout helps improve thought processes in all age groups, from senior executives to schoolchildren. Since there is not enough room to cover all these options, you should pick those that serve your interests and circumstances. Here are some recommended individual exercises for your consideration or order them through MindBodySeries.com:

- "Air conducting" a fantasy orchestra
- Drumming a consistent pattern on a drum
- Playing a musical instrument
- Singing
- Slow dancing to gentle music
- Swimming laps
- Tai chi
- Yoga
- Walking

## Team Exercises

Team exercises provide additional benefits by stimulating the brain's problem-solving, memory, and reactive coordination abilities. Even a game of poker stimulates your brain dramatically. (If it doesn't, I'd like to play some serious poker with you some time.)

More physical sports like table tennis or basketball benefit your reactive coordination. And if you win, you get mood elevation too! But remember, anytime you are getting the exercise your body and mind so desperately need, you are already a winner.

The areas of the brain affected include the frontal lobes, the cerebellum, the temporal lobe, the parietal motor regions, and the occipital lobe. The temporal lobe handles social relations, emotional states, and memory, all of which are put to work in these exercises.

Some great group exercises to try include:

• Dancing with a partner

• Hiking in groups

• Playing a musical instrument in a band

• Singing with a group

• Table tennis

• Tennis

• Volleyball

## The Power of Rhythm and Harmony

Music has a powerful effect on our emotions and on our brains, sometimes for the better, sometimes for the worse. Simply put, the brain reacts to music. That's why we often feel inspired, saddened, or just pumped up by music. There is a definite difference between your brain's response to a death march and a parade march. That is because different kinds of music affect different areas of the brain. Gospel music that seems to trigger hopeful emotions stimulates the amygdala, a very deep center in the brain. That is why those who are strongly affected by gospel music might be motivated to seek a higher purpose for their lives. Interestingly, sexually stimulating "mood" music also affects the lower cortex.

My clinic has developed a set of drum rhythms on CD that are designed to aid in reconnections and to orient the brain as quickly as possible. They start with a basic heartbeat and progress in complexity, much like the brain increases its complex patterning. They are ideal for the PTSD healing process, which can actually begin while in the hyperbaric chambers. If interested, anyone can purchase them by called the PNP Center in Lewisville, Texas (972-434-5454) or order them through MindBodySeries.com.

• Brain Orientation Rhythms #1: The basic heartbeat everyone uses to orient to life.

- Brain Orientation Rhythms #2: The Steady Life Rhythms of Joy

- Brain Orientation Rhythms #3: The Evolvement of Complex Emotions

- Brain Orientation Rhythms #4: The Awareness of the Emerging Self

- Brain Orientation Rhythms #5: The Coordination of Differences

- Brain Orientation Rhythms #6: The Connections between our Roots and Divinities

- Brain Orientation Rhythms #7: The Global Self

Sometimes when a patient is stressed, panicked, or even in a rage, I ask them to hum or sing a song. After a few minutes, the brain responds in fascinating ways. Sometimes a person will find a melody and rhythm that comes out of the blue. They behave happier and become optimistic, breaking out of depression and anxiety.

What is your power song? What tune might bring your brain into a more powerful state? You can't sing, you say? Not true. We all have the ability to create rhythms and melodies. Don't put pressure on yourself and judge the way your voice sounds compared to Celine Dion; just let it out naturally for your own pleasure. Do it in the shower (very good acoustics in there) or alone in your bedroom where you feel safe. This may be the most enjoyable therapy you ever undertake. So, fire up the iTunes, head for the music store or even the neighborhood library's loaner collection, and find the song that sets your mind and your heart free. There are some types of music I don't recommend for this, though. Avoid music that has an angry or depressing message. For example, although I was once a country and western amateur singer and guitar picker, many of those songs are just depressing to listen to without getting dragged down emotionally.

## Mental Exercise

A most effective way to reconnect the brain, of course, is to exercise the mind. The mind needs a focus in order to coordinate itself for action. You can't orient yourself in a vacuum or else you will lose yourself in chaos. Nerve endings in the idle brain begin to lose connections with major centers and receptor sites fall away, blocking the passage of neuron transmissions. The best way to prevent problems is to keep exercising the brain with mental challenges.

Just as physical exercise generates strength in various

parts of the body, mental exercises build strength in the exercised parts of the brain. As we previously discussed, nerve fibers (neurons) collect where there is action and stimulation. Individual mental exercises generally affect the three areas of the frontal (executive region), temporal (memory), and occipital (visual imagery) lobes.

I have assembled some mind-exercise games for you, including a few from the American Mensa library for your consideration. Mensa is an organization for those who rank in the top 2 percent of the population intellectually. Its mission is to foster human intelligence. I have been the supervisory psychologist for this fine organization for a number of years. Its members are some of the most gracious people I've met, and, needless to say, they are pretty sharp cookies too. Mensa members love to play mental games to stimulate their minds. Here are some of their favorites:

- 3 Stones
- 10 Days in Africa
- Abalone
- Apples to Apples
- Avalam
- Basari
- Blokus

- Bollox
- Brainstrain
- The Bridges of Shangri-La
- Char
- Chung Toi
- Cityscape

- Clue: The Great Museum Caper
- Continuo
- Cube Checkers
- Curses!
- DAO
- Doubles Wild
- Down Fall
- Duo
- Dvonn
- Farook
- Finish Lines
- Fire & Ice
- Fluxx
- The Great Dalmuti

## Puzzles

- *Great Word Search Puzzles for Kids*, Mark Danan
- *Mensa Book of Words*, Abbie Salny, PhD
- *Mensa Genius ABC Quiz Book*, Alan Stillson
- *Mensa Quiz a Day*, Abbie Salny, PhD, et al.
- *Mensa Think Smart*, Abbie Salny, PhD

## Interpersonal Games

- Bridge
- Bingo
- Charades
- Checkers
- Chess
- Clue
- Poker

# Blue Light

The final method for reorienting your brain may be the most interesting one. This might come as a shock to some, but different shades of light stimulate the brain. A very inexpensive way for your brain to get oriented (especially in the morning) is to expose yourself to blue light. Research clearly shows that our frontal lobes get quite excited in response to blue light, improving our organizational skills and memory.

My clinic has been recommending blue light for children and adults with ADHD and PTSD for years with excellent results. All you have to do is go down to your friendly hardware store and buy a twenty-five- or forty-watt blue light bulb and plug it into a lamp. Have the blue light on in your room for about ten or fifteen minutes and you are tuning your brain for the day.

I have no reason why blue is better than red or green, but the research is consistent that blue activates higher attention factors of the brain. Maybe it is due to it being the shortest wavelength, or maybe it's because blue is the color of the sky. No matter what the reason, it simply works.

# Final Comment

Brain orientation is a critical phase in the Compass RESET process for PTSD rehabilitation. And it is probably the scariest. As the brain heals, it grows into more awareness, which may mean more confusion and distrust. It may be like coming out of the fog and finding yourself in a war and you don't know which side you are supposed to be on.

You will also find that there is little that you enjoy in life, especially those things in which you once found comfort and happiness. That is part of the disorientation so common in brain injury. Unfortunately your brain pleasure centers haven't oriented themselves with labels you understand, which leaves you without relief from stress and on the edge of depression.

This situation can create problems on those nights when you feel the loneliest and without understanding. What I want to do is to remind you that a better end is coming. The darkest hours are often just before the dawn, but dawn does indeed arrive. So, please hold on through this tough part, because the best parts, in the next steps, will soon be within your reach.

# CHAPTER FIVE

# Step Four: Relinquishing Fear and Rage

Jose sat looking into space for a long time, and I wondered what was racing through his mind. He had been a patient of mine for about two months, and we had gotten to know each other pretty well, so I was concerned with what might be going on. He didn't seem to hear my inquiries, and we were not in a "session," just drinking coffee and casually chatting with a group. As if he was not talking to anyone in particular, he began to tell a story that I will never forget.

"The commander kept telling me to drive, just drive and not stop. I heard the thumps and had to keep telling myself they were just bags, not children, just bags. It was the hardest thing I ever did, keep driving, just driving. I knew the commander had his gun to my head, but it made no difference because I knew it was up to me. I was so scared, so I kept driving," Jose said.

Then he stopped as if waking from a dream and looked at me. Jose was a shy guy, so I thought he was going to stop, but he didn't. It was like he was finally sharing something he had kept inside for too long. He continued, "You see, I was driving the lead supply truck, and they made it look like there were children lying down across the road, and if we stopped, they would attack us from the sides." He paused for about a minute as he drank another sip of coffee.

"You see, it was me and the commander and we had to go on or everyone would die. It was bad, real bad. The noise was deafening with flashes of light from everywhere. I kept telling myself these were not children, just bags, but they looked like children, but they were not. Sometimes I heard children cry in the night and I wondered, did I kill them or were they really bags?"

Another pause while he contemplated his words and focused on me, "I was so scared I would have done anything, even kill my child maybe. That is what scares me most. What am I capable of? Do you think I would come to that, doc?"

I looked him in the face, deep in his eyes, and gently said, "No, I don't. You were scared and felt responsible for something you didn't do. Those were only bags. The mind is just confusing you about what you could have done. I know that. You know that. Everyone knows that."

"Do you really believe that, Doc?"

"Yes, I do."

"Then why am I still scared? I think I know that, but even when you say it, or anyone else says that, I must not believe it because I am still scared."

"Because fear is not rational. It is buried deep inside your brain and can't be talked over and beat out of you. You are trying to make sense of it, of what you are feeling, explaining to yourself your best theory, but the fact remains that you are scared and don't know what to do about it. Am I right?"

Jose was shaken by my words. "Doc, does that mean it will never go away?"

"No, you can make it go away, and if you want to do that, we can do it now."

Jose was stunned. He did not believe me, but he was cautiously excited. "How?"

I pulled out the BAUD, a little device about the size of a cigarette package that emits sounds like bees (which are the frequencies that the brain makes), and had him sit directly in front of me across the table. "Here, put these earphones in your ears. When I turn on the noise, I want you to turn up the volume as high as you are comfortable. I want your brain to pay attention to that noise and drown out everything else."

When he had set the volume level, he looked at me and I turned off the device. "What I want you to do now, and I know this may be hard, is to go back and imagine that situation. What I am trying to see is what your arousal frequency is. Our brains typically have a frequency that accounts for our anxieties and fears. And everybody's is different. So as you are focusing on your fearful situation, I want you to turn this knob slowly, and when your fearful emotions get worse, stop and show me the frequency when they got worse."

As Jose closed his eyes and turned the frequency knob, he concentrated on his emotional levels. The peak frequency was apparent because he began to sweat and breathe hard. He opened his eyes and said, "This is it."

"Good, now continue to concentrate on that situation and turn this knob until the emotion dissolves away. You can feel the emotion being disrupted."

He closed his eyes for concentration as he slowly turned the disruptor knob. About twenty seconds passed. The results were obvious even before he told us because he began to grin and smile. As he opened his eyes, he was markedly relaxed and everyone could see the relief on his face. "Wow, what happened?"

I quickly asked him to just relax by listening to the frequencies he just set and taking long breaths for four minutes. At the end of that period, I asked him to do a very difficult thing: laugh at the scary images he held. All of the group joined in a forced laughter as he kept listening to the BAUD and laughing at his situation, as if he were laughing at the power the situation held over him for so long.

Fast forward six months. Jose has not had another fear attack or nightmare since and has found peace.

For those who suffer from PTSD, one of the most common symptoms is a life controlled by crippling fear, which often results in the victim being consumed by rage. The next step of PTSD recovery involves understanding why this fear and rage occurs in the brain and how to overcome it.

# Defining Fear

Emotions such as fear play essential roles in our lives and are present as the deepest instinctual response to potential danger. These instinctual reactions are rooted deep inside the brain and serve to protect us. When a person senses fear, the brain reacts by activating two systems: the sympathetic system to alert the body and the parasympathetic system to restore and heal. When the sympathetic system is aroused, certain areas of the brain, called the amygdala and hypothalamus, become activated and biochemicals, such as adrenaline and a stress hormone, cortisol, are released into the bloodstream. These changes are felt in the body as:

- Rapid heart rate
- Increased blood pressure
- Tightening of muscles
- Sharpened or redirected senses

• Dilation of the pupils (to let in more light)

• Increased sweating

It is important to understand that such changes do not happen in our bodies because of rational thought; instead they are activated by the instinctive fear response, which resides in a different part of the brain. Because this response is instinctual, it is not very adaptive. It carries with it a huge power over our sense of peace of mind and prohibits other parts of the brain from functioning effectively. It can affect the parasympathetic system's ability to slow down and nourish our activated organs, alert our immune systems, heal our wounds, and help us feel safe and comfortable.

At the brain level, there is a specific area, known as the rostral cingulate, which engages the brain in finding solutions to the fear stimulations and creating resolutions. At least, that is what is supposed to happen. But if we allow the high level of fear to persist at all times, we hurt ourselves. We become vulnerable to disease because our immune system doesn't work, we don't react appropriately to the reality we are in, and we don't make good choices. We can be crippled both emotionally and physically. And it can lead to rage.

# The Rage Phase

Rage is a common reaction in those with PTSD, especially the soldiers, because it is a behavior to defend oneself. Rage is an irrational attempt to relieve fear by attacking someone else. It can be effective in a battle situation, but if that rage is used in our everyday lives, it simply doesn't work.

Rage is an extension of the *reflexive fighting response* (RFR). The RFR is an automatic response to stress in which you attack anyone close to you when stress increases. I ran an experiment when I was in graduate school in which I put two rats in a cage together with a floor that sent electricity to the feet of the rats. (Please note this was not enough of an electrical charge to cause harm to the rats.) Whenever I would push the button to send a mild charge, the rats would automatically fight. Fear triggers a rage response.

The trigger does not have to be electric shock. It could be heat, cold, overcrowding, or anything else that could induce stress. This seems to be a universal response among all animals, even humans. This RFR principle shows us that stress is the culprit of rage, and therefore learning how to manage this stress is key.

# Assessment

So how do you know if your fear and rage are normal, or out of control? If you are hurting others or are aware of your fear, you of course don't need this test—you know the answer already. But your situation may be less certain—there is a level of denial that often protects us from seeing ourselves as cruel and hurtful.

This short checklist will help you determine your levels of fear and rage. Check off those characteristics you see in yourself or someone you are worried about:

___ Do you have doubts about your ability to control your fear or anger?

___ Do you lose control of your temper and say things or behave in a way that is beyond your own standards of safe conduct?

___ Do you try to hide your anger, only to have it explode at times?

___ Do you avoid people or situations in which you might lose control?

___ Do you harm animals or children?

___ Do you obsess over your fear of losing control of outbursts?

___ Do you forget about your outbursts and rages, even if someone tells you about them?

___ Do you have nightmares every night?

___ Are you afraid of yourself?

___ Do you worry you will lose control and be deprived of your family?

___ Do you feel like a monster?

___ Do you feel flooded with memories of being extremely afraid and unable to respond?

___ Do you want to flee from your living circumstances and hide so that your anxieties can subside?

___ Do you find your body in a highly anxious state (heart racing, hands sweating, fast breathing, etc.) and you are not aware of the reasons for it?

___ Do you ruin objects or act aggressively when you feel emotional (punching holes in walls, throwing objects out of anger, driving aggressively, etc.)?

If you checked off two or more of the items, you have a fear issue, and you may have rage problems. This phase of the Compass RESET Program may be the most rewarding of the phases because it will put you in charge of your emotions and brain functioning. You will discover your strengths of self-control. It will give you the coping measures that can help. Let's look at each of these methods and how they can help overcome the fear and rage that comprise one of the most difficult parts of PTSD.

## Methods of Desensitization

The major step for PTSD patients is to disconnect their automatic fear response from emotional triggers. This process is called "systematic desensitization," and it teaches you to develop a process in which the arousal system of stress is separated from increasing stress triggers, one by one.

Let's say you have a fear of heights that you wanted to dispose of because you work on the ninety-ninth floor of a building. The first step would be to develop a hierarchy of fears, starting with the item you fear the least. In our example, you would list the following fears:

1. *Opening the door of the building*

2. *Looking at the elevator*

3. *Walking into the elevator*

4. *Experiencing the elevator rise*

5. *Getting off the elevator*

6. *Looking at the window overlooking the city*

7. *Looking down at ground level from the window*

The therapist would then put you in a relaxed state and begin describing your first step, opening the door, and so on. Anytime you begin to feel anxious, you would signal the therapist by raising your finger, and then you would start over from the beginning. You continue these steps until you achieve the last step. Then you must go through all the steps in reality and accomplish the task.

In another approach to desensitization, you imagine your worst fears or even experience them directly until the fear just exhausts itself. This one is scary because you have to wait until the fear subsides, which might take weeks. To break it off early will cause greater fears. In our example, this would mean that you would have to either imagine or actually look at the ground level from the window ninety-nine stories high until you weren't afraid anymore.

There are two issues with these methods. The first is that both of them were developed for irrational beliefs. It may be irrational to freak out when driving over high bridges, but I would question if it's irrational to be afraid when there are bullets coming at you, or a menacing group of people are racing at you with the objective of erasing your existence from this world. Fear does have a healthy reason for being and to try to convince the brain there is no reason to be afraid would make a person crazy.

The second issue is that these methods are based on rational processes, and as I have explained, the fear associated with PTSD does not come from the rational part of the brain. It is deeper than a problem to be solved. But the most important piece of information is that desensitization does not work on a reliable basis. I have talked with soldiers who are in these therapies for a year. That means for me they aren't working.

## What Does Work: The BAUD

When I was working as clinical professor of orthopedic surgery at Southwestern Medical School in Dallas, my specialty was chronic back and neck pain. I was put in charge of our failures in spinal surgery. In these cases patients had serious problems of chronic pain—pain medicine did not work and could be addictive, physical therapy yielded nothing but more pain, and even bed rest made it worse for them.

I jumped at the chance to prove my psychological skills and failed at every attempt I made. I tried hypnosis, I did intensive psychotherapy at the underlying reasons, I tried confrontation. I tried everything I knew and finally faced the fact that I knew nothing about how to help these people.

Finally, I attended a workshop by Dr. Michael Harner on how "medicine men," or shamans, cured the ills of pain without our gracious allotment of modern medicine. He told me I needed to "learn the drum." After some instruction in basic drumming techniques, I was ready to test this approach.

I gathered my twenty patients in a room and told them

I was going to beat the drum and we would see what happened. I started beating on my drum at about four to five beats per second. I expected half of them to revolt against the sound, but after twenty minutes, they were all still there. To my surprise, about a fourth of them reported their pain had completely gone for the time being, and all of them reported a significant decrease in their pain.

Later research based on this experience showed that persistent drumming at certain rates caused the brain frequency to shift into a lower level, increasing relaxation and decreasing stress. Further exploration by others showed an increase in endorphin activity levels and a lowering of stress hormones. This was an exciting breakthrough, but the potential to help others was limited by one's physical ability to beat a drum more than eight beats a minute.

To solve this problem, I partnered with an engineer to create what I call the bioacoustical utilization device, or BAUD. Much like how Charles Goodyear accidentally discovered the secret of making vulcanized rubber by adding sulfur and heating it, I have been guided by a similar force in understanding the BAUD's nature and success.

In simple terms, the BAUD is an electronic device that simulates the positive effects of drumming. You can refer to the way I used it with Jose at the beginning of this chapter. You find the frequency of your fears by imagining your fearful situation and turning the frequency knob that raises the pitch (and frequency) of the "buzz." When your emotions escalate at a certain sound frequency, you have found the specific arousal level for that particular fear.

Then you turn a knob that separates the frequency into two frequencies, one for each ear, and the sounds will begin to disrupt each other. It is when you discover that the emotional fear you are experiencing has been disrupted that you are disrupting the fear response in your brain. It is my theory that the two frequencies create a third one by the overlap, and it is this third wave that stimulates the parasympathetic frequency for your brain.

Essentially, by shutting down a frequency that your brain has been using inappropriately and resetting the frequency at a lower one that is conducive to relaxation instead of panic, you are shifting the pattern to a more adaptable one.

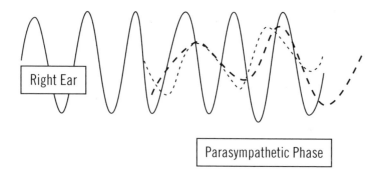

Frequencies of right and left ear resulting in a third interference wave.

There are 1,350 BAUD devices being used throughout the world, and we have received over eight hundred positive reports. There have been three *Dr. Phil* shows in which the BAUD device was used and produced positive results within forty minutes. The applications were done backstage without cameras or public knowledge in order to preserve the process. An organized clinical research project is underway in which eighty-six subjects around the world were shown to have immediate results. If you have any interest, look at the website, www.BAUDenergetics. com (check the professional link for illustrations).

While the success of the BAUD is exciting, it is a new development, and thus it might not be the easiest method to work into your recovery right away. If this is the case for you, the following are other effective methods you can use to address your fear and rage problems.

## Biofeedback Approaches

Biofeedback is a method that helps your body to relax so that you can cope with any threat you may have. It is a method in which you train your body, especially the stress behaviors, to relax.

A computer is used to measure some of those stress measures, such as heart rate, blood pressure, muscle tension, blood flow restriction, skin sweating, and brain functions that relate to stress.

Selecting your most serious stressors, you train your body by observing via the computer how it responds to different approaches. For example, you might discover that breathing in certain patterns brings down your blood pressure or relaxes your muscles. Or you may find that when you focus on your hand relaxing, your shoulder muscles relax as well. By training your body to relax, you can learn new coping skills for your stresses. The Biofeedback Society has provided numerous research studies to demonstrate the credibility of this approach.

There is a more direct biofeedback approach using the electroencephalogram (EEG) that measures brain frequencies. By observing the reactions to your stress triggers and using various methods (like breathing and visualizing), you can teach your brain new ways to react. It is like teaching your body to wiggle your ears by looking at them in the mirror. This is the root of brain plasticity, where you are actually modifying the brain. If you are interested in this approach, contact www.bica.org.

## The emWave

The emWave device is essentially a computer that does three functions that can teach you how to relax. First, it computes your heart rate variability from your heart pulse. Heart rate variability is how steadily your heart pumps—the more steady, the more relaxed.

The next step is rather remarkable. Based on your pulse rate, it calculates the breathing pattern you need to have in order to become more relaxed and shows this pace with a light that goes up and down. If you follow this light pattern with your breath, exhaling as it goes down and inhaling as it goes up, you will automatically adjust your heart rate to your breathing in such a way that you become physically and emotionally relaxed. It is like training yourself to relax through customized breathing patterns.

The third step is that it indicates to you if you are successfully relaxing by another light that goes from red (not good) to blue (good) to green (very good). It even keeps score of how well you're doing. This device has been very helpful in teaching people to learn the relaxation response.

Another brain plasticity application is evident by this technique. By teaching your body to breathe and coordinate with your heart rate, you are sending messages to your brain via your nerves. There are many more nerve fibers going from your heart to the brain than vice versa, so by using this method, you can affect changes quickly for relaxation.

## Using Smells

We often use a technique involving smells for situations in which we need to provide a mental shield against the rush of stress, especially rage. It is quick and inexpensive to do.

First you have to choose a smell that is powerful and positive, or at least emotionally neutral. Many people choose flowers, which are the best choice if available. I also suggest going to a health-food store and picking up an essential oil (a highly concentrated aroma that comes in a little jar). They have a variety of smells, so you can try them out and make a selection. I have found that clove, peppermint, and eucalyptus are the winners, but honeysuckle and jasmine are also good candidates.

Rub a small amount into the palm of your hand. Now think of your stressful situation. Bring your emotions high and, at the peak, and take a big whiff of your chosen scent. Fill your whole head with the smell and then notice that your stress emotions are immediately shattered.

The reason your fear or rage emotion goes away is because the smell sensation goes directly to the brain and cuts off all other messages going on, at least for a while. Like the BAUD, the smell disrupts all processing on an emotional level. The brain is just wired to do this. This disruption doesn't last for more than an hour, but it does offer the opportunity to make better choices for constructive behavioral responses. People have used this method to deal very successfully with their rage and excessive worrying.

## Cognitive-Behavioral Approaches

Other approaches ask you to challenge your fears with some rules. These rules help your mind by highlighting the emotional investments we place on the underlying values of our beliefs, which can cause high anxiety. After all, the challenges we build ourselves are often the most difficult to get through.

For example, suppose you had a basic belief that you have to deal with all your problems by yourself or you would be weak and dependent. (This is the classic PTSD profile for soldiers.) But now you have been a victim of something you need some help with. Every time you ask for help, your inner mind ridicules you and makes you feel worthless and insufficient. By confronting the belief that asking for help is senseless, you can rid yourself of the deep-seated self-criticism that might be sabotaging you.

But it's not easy. Many of your damaging beliefs are very deep in your subconscious and have to be clarified in steps. A cognitive-behavioral treatment is one that is based on the idea that psychological problems arise as a result of the way in which we interpret or evaluate situations, thoughts, feelings, or behaviors.

Let's say you almost drown, or even lose consciousness, in an accident, and you can remember the feeling of suffocation and the near death of your body. The last feeling you had was terror, and you could imagine losing your life and family. Because of the fear, you take extraordinary steps to avoid swimming in pools and lakes. This avoidance behavior may work most of the time, unless, for example, you are invited for a cruise or you find yourself thinking about having to go near water for a special occasion. Because you harbor the fear, you will be anxious about the subject and/or you may sabotage your chances for a fuller and richer life.

Worries like these can be quite taxing, and unfortunately we really cannot avoid our thoughts. Our energy resources can only stretch so far, and such stress can actually lower our intelligence on other issues. Avoidance and denial may not work as well for thoughts or memories that are upsetting, like those that occur in PTSD. People with PTSD may try more extreme strategies such as drinking or using drugs. Using substances may help someone forget about something briefly. However, the thoughts just return, usually more intensely. In addition, the substance used will just cause a whole host of other problems.

Cognitive-behavioral psychotherapy has been the primary approach that has been shown to "work." Brain-mapping has shown it actually changes the brain (brain plasticity), and behaviors become significantly more appropriate. I strongly recommend using this mental health professional specialty, based on its high level of research applications and efficacy. To begin this treatment, seek out the psychologists in your area who are trained in this specialty (their names are available through state boards for licensed psychologists).

## General Approach of CBT

The concept for cognitive-behavioral therapy (CBT) mentioned previously is that if people can change how they evaluate their environment or thoughts and feelings, anxiety and avoidance may be reduced, improving mood and overall quality of life. You use two basic processes: self-monitoring and cognitive restructuring.

In the self-monitoring phases, you write down as much as you can about the fear-inducing aspects you can describe. Then with the help of a therapist, you confront the situation with some rules, such as:

- Is the situation or worry real? Are the fears really justified? In our example, the fear of water and drowning can be confronted with the reality that there are very few actual situations in which you can drown if you know how to swim and take care to protect yourself and your family from the risks. Yes, there are some risks, so it is important to educate yourself; however, the probability is very low in any case.

- Is the situation life-threatening? For the ordinary situation, no, and excessive worrying is not necessary.

- Is it to your advantage in life to worry about the situation? No, it is not to your advantage to worry about this event.

Once these evaluations are identified, you can learn more appropriate emotions. For example, you can teach yourself to have reality checks, and only become worried when there is clear evidence a danger should worry you. Or you can find someone you trust to look for danger zones, and only allow yourself to worry when one is spotted. This process is called cognitive restructuring.

# Diaries and Journaling

Finally, psychological science has revealed that one of the worst things you can do for victims of trauma is to require them to tell their story over and over again. Many times, victims of traumatic situations, such as airplane crashes and automobile accidents, suffer from well-meaning people asking them to repeatedly describe the horrible events they just went through with the false assumption that they need to "get it out."

Nothing could be further from the truth. One of the reasons people have to adjust to a traumatic event is that it is so different from any other event in their lives that their minds cannot grasp all of the experience yet. They are reeling from just going through bizarre circumstances that are like nothing they have experienced before. And here someone is, in their face, trying to get them to reexperience that event, making it more difficult for the mind to understand.

This is especially true for grief and loss. I get very angry when I see some reporter sticking a microphone in the nose of someone who is on the edge of shock and asking some stupid question like, "And how does it feel to lose your children and husband to the fire that just engulfed your house and all of your precious possessions?"

Adjusting your mind to tragic circumstances is hard, and it takes time for things to get sorted out. To rush it is to create dangerous shortcuts. It is always better to allow for the healing process to occur naturally. For that reason, journaling can be very helpful.

Journaling is simply writing down your thoughts every day as they come to you. I would recommend setting aside a time of day, usually thirty minutes, in a quiet place and just let it happen. This is not a contest. Make it a pleasant experience. The mind will reveal what you need to know when it can be integrated with everything else. It might be a plan to understand and appreciate some aspects of the process before your mind can tolerate new information.

I remember trying to come to terms with my father's death when I was a teenager. I first had to grieve our relationship and what I had wanted it to be and what it wasn't before I could begin to grieve his loss. Then I had to come to terms with his limitations and my own denial of them. I learned a lot from that journaling.

## The Process in Perspective

This chapter has been about releasing the burdens of fear, anger, and loss. These transitions are more than just acts of will or accidental. In this chapter scientific methods have been discussed. Using sonic stimulation, as with the BAUD, the brain can shift from stress to relaxation, and along with that shift comes peace and rational processing. Training your body and mind into more adaptive responses through biofeedback, or correcting the mind's faulty logical system through cognitive methods, also bring positive results. Even more naturalistic methods, such as using smells and writing for your own wisdom are very effective. You can take action to unburden yourself so that you can fly again in your heart. This is never simple, but full of surprises and adventure. That is what life is all about.

And it is with this release of the weight and confusion that you take the next step into what will be the beginning of the rest of your life. These steps cannot be taken without a plan or a program like the Compass RESET Program. Otherwise you might find yourself circling back to where you began. That is the focus of the next chapter in your life.

CHAPTER SIX

# Step Five: Creating a New Beginning

Ted was scared and angry about his homecoming, even though it had been three months ago. It was not about the celebration and how glad people were to see him; rather, he was disturbed because they didn't see him as different. Everyone seemed to see him as exactly the same person who left for war the year before. It was as if the months of being in hell had not changed him. He couldn't blame them because they didn't know what he had gone through, and, of course, he wasn't going to tell them. To tell the awful truth would cause more shame for him than the high praise they were giving him. He had done some things that no one should ever know, and he expected all of the other troops would keep the silence as well.

Ted had left behind his wife, who was pregnant with their first child, his parents, brothers, sisters, and friends to do a tour of duty in the war. Ted described this group as having all the love a family could possibly have. The tour was unexpected, but he wanted to do his duty as he had promised his country. Although he showed his sadness in leaving, he was excited to go and was ready. After all, he was in the marines and felt the pride of his corps.

His family had known him for many years—or at least they thought they knew him—but when Ted returned home after his tour, he had changed into another person and no one noticed. No one could imagine all the human misery he had seen. They could not possibly have a clue of the torment he felt as he prayed for life and prepared to die at the same time. They could see the missing fingers and foot that had been ripped away by the explosion of the bomb on the side of the road, but they could not see the much worse damage that he carried within. He acted as if the injuries and Purple Heart award meant little more than just getting in the way of his goals, but in a way he wanted his family to understand the shock and recognize that he was not a whole body anymore. (No marine will ever discount the importance of a Purple Heart; however, in large part because of their training, they will instead talk about the other guy who didn't make it home, or who was hurt much worse. They are trained to deflect praise or recognition and focus on their team and buddies.) Ted was lucky, maybe, but he was not whole anymore.

And he was angry, very angry, when people blew it off with "you're lucky that you are still alive" comments.

Yes, he had survived, but what had survived of his life? What was left? He continued to play the role, as he had always done, of being the strong and confident one. He was the oldest brother and therefore carried the family burden. If he let down his guard, he would let down the whole family. He was surprised when he realized that one of the things he most desired to do was cry. He didn't know why, but he thought it might demonstrate just how different he was and that he did not want to and could not carry the family morale any longer. He was not the same person they once believed in, and if he could just leave, he would. "It was so f——g hard," he wanted to say to them, so much that he even dreamed about it.

The feeling got worse when someone, usually his father or wife, would ask him when he was going to get back into life and do the things he had wanted to do. He clenched his jaw so much he had broken two teeth, and his headaches were enough to send him to bed for half a day.

Ted's marriage was also in decline, and he knew it. His baby, a little girl, had been born while he was on duty, and when he returned, he did the usual daddy things, like holding her, trying to be attentive, and appreciating his wife for keeping the home fires burning while he was away at war.

But this was an act. Deep down he was deeply distracted and very confused. He hated to admit to himself that his feelings for his baby and wife were not what he expected them to be. They were not a priority for him, and he hated himself for that. He left excited about having a child with the woman he loved. He had spent months dreaming of all the things he was going to do with his baby and how amazing it was going to be when they were together as a family. In fact, this was part of what got him through the many months of fighting. Now he saw both his wife and baby as responsibilities and even burdens preventing him from doing what he really wanted to do. His lack of deep emotions for them turned into self-hatred that he could not admit to himself and certainly not to anyone who knew him.

What he wanted to do was run, to escape the past and the constant demands of family life. To be free. He had done his duty; now he wanted to be done with it all. If he could, he would buy a motorcycle and roam the countryside, grow a long beard, and live in the same clothes every day for a year. He definitely wanted to do all this, but knew his mind would only constantly remind him of his duties at home and his obligation to be the person everyone expected him to be.

In many ways Ted actually wanted his grogginess and poor memory, because he could likely enjoy not knowing what he knows now: that life is not what it used to be. Ted did get past the torment I just described, but it took some long hours of talk with a counselor and some reorganization of his life plans. He went through some scary moments. He divorced his wife and married her again. He left home multiple times just to get some space, but luckily he did not go to the bottle for relief. He feels joy now, but he is a lot different than even he thought he had the potential to be.

## Starting Over

Ted is like the thousands of other returning soldiers or victims of traumatic events who immediately recognize that "home" is not a place you can return to easily. Home may be the same as you left it, but everything else about you may be different. Your physical body may be different; it may be missing parts or scarred up or simply older. Your mind has lived through the long periods of time away at war, work, or the event that changed you. It takes a lot of awareness to see that the change in you is permanent, and if you don't come to terms with it, you will always be a stranger to yourself. You have to push the RESET button.

After all the brain healing and reconnecting and working through fear and rage, the next steps come down to who you are, and who you will be. Your "home" must now be redesigned from the ground up. Your life must be redesigned from the ground up. And it may be different from the life you envisioned before the events that caused your PTSD occurred—after all, you are quite a different person now. But if you are to succeed in your recovery, you must face this challenge.

What you need to realize is that you go away and you come back, but the only thing you come back with is your name. You need to create a plan to start all over and recognize that this chapter in your life could be over. If you look back on your life, you will probably see that it was a series of chapters, like a book, and this is the first blank page opening where your new adventures are to be written.

Psychologists break down life into stages, such as infancy, childhood, preteens, adolescence, young adulthood, middle age, and the elder years. Each stage has its own beginnings and endings, with certain tasks and developmental skills required of each. For example, during infancy the development of bonds with parents occur, and the infant learns ways of survival, such as eating and finding security. The childhood stage is characterized by learning the rules of culture and developing skills, while the preteen years are marked by discovering social rules and establishing friendships. Teens carry the heavy load of developing adult skills, such as relationships with the opposite sex.

This chapter may be called the "post-PTSD" chapter. You are creating the next chapter of your life.

# The Skills You Carry

This does not mean, of course, that you forget everything about your former life. You have talents learned in your earlier stages that you will use in developing your new life. You may want to take a moment to list the strengths you can transfer into this stage. Remember that it will be your strengths that will give you your greatest resources, not your limitations.

For example, some of the strengths Ted listed were:

- Ability to talk to people
- Ability to set goals and accomplish them without distractions
- Strong organizational skills among people
- Strong leadership skills
- Willingness to listen and help someone
- Good looks

Ted felt that his skills centered on working with people, so he directed the next chapter of his life toward the management of people. He went back to school for a two-year degree in management and found a satisfying career along those lines.

You may find your way back to your original ideas of what you wanted your life to be. Contemplate a choice as opposed to just going with the flow. You may make a dozen lists of your strengths and even ask your friends and family to name a few you don't recognize yourself. For this moment in this chapter, I would ask you to write down seven of your strengths:

1. _____

2. _____

3. _____

4. _____

5. _____

6. _____

7. _____

## Looking Backward

I am now going to ask you to do an exercise that may sound scary and even morbid, but it will definitely help you in the long run.

Fast forward to the end of your life. Imagine you are either on your deathbed or at your funeral, looking down from a high place. While you may be enjoying watching the scene below, I want you to think about all the things you hope that you have accomplished during your lifetime.

Ted listed the following and was willing to share them with anyone who was going through this process:

- Was a productive worker
- Provided for my family
- Led a good religious life
- Did not go to jail
- Had a good family life I could be proud of
- Provided good leadership to people who needed it
- Took care of my parents

Now it's your turn. What are seven things you hope you can achieve during your lifetime? You may have already accomplished some of these.

1. _____

2. _____

3. _____

4. _____

5. _____

6. _____

7. _____

Before we proceed, please take some time and arrange them from most important to least important. Now limit your list to five things you want to do, which may be part of your original seven or may be new ones. You can take your time doing this; don't rush it. This is very heavy stuff to think about, because you may be evaluating yourself from time to time.

Taking the five hopes you placed in order, determine at least three steps you will be taking in the next week or the next month to accomplish these goals. You will be taking steps the rest of your life probably, but let's get started now.

Goal #1: _____ Step #1: _____

Step #2: _____

Step #3: _____

Goal #2: _____ Step #1: _____

Step #2: _____

Step #3: _____

Goal #3: _____ Step #1: _____

                                    Step #2: _____

                                    Step #3: _____

Goal #4: _____ Step #1: _____

                                    Step #2: _____

                                    Step #3: _____

Goal #5: _____ Step #1: _____

                                    Step #2: _____

                                    Step #3: _____

This is your to-do list for your life and an outline of the most important things you have in mind. But it is not a rigid list. There will be opportunities you didn't know existed that will appear, and you always want to be flexible enough to consider another path. But at the same time, you don't want to jump to every new idea that pops up along the way. That is the reason you want a list to start with as the higher value for yourself.

## From Doing to Being

The last exercise was focused on what you hope to do or accomplish during your lifetime. But as all of us know we are human "beings," not human "doings." The next set of questions is what you want to *be* in your lifetime.

This description may sound a little absurd, but the way you are as a being is more important than what you do. You can be a millionaire or a janitor, and it would make no difference if you were a "being" who respected yourself. Remember that all the research is consistent in the findings that you are going to be happy and unhappy in your lifetime for about the same amount of time, regardless of money, power, or profession. So if you are counting on a lifetime of living happy all the time, you will be surprised and disappointed. Even Cinderella is unhappy sometimes because those glass slippers hurt her feet and have caused arthritis.

After a few days of thinking about this, go back to the vision you had of the end of your life in the previous exercise. Make a list of what you would have liked to be during your lifetime.

Ted shared these with me and you as examples:

- A generous person
- A religious person
- An honest person
- A good father
- A good provider

You may notice some overlap in the two lists, and that is normal. As long as you have the concept of the difference between "doing" and "being" you are doing it correctly.

1. _____

2. _____

3. _____

4. _____

5. _____

As we did above, arrange these "being" states into a priority list from most important to least important. Since these traits hold a lot of value for an individual, there may be more than five in your list, and they may be very difficult to rank. You may have some points that are tied in their rankings, or you may be able to blend some together. Take your time with this, as these may serve as your guideposts along the journey to recovery.

As you list your new "being" states, make a list of behaviors and attitudes you will be focusing on to serve them. This is your "walk the talk" time.

1. Example: Being a          Behavior/attitude:   patient
   good father              Behavior/attitude:   aware of being a
                                                 model

                           Behavior/attitude:   _____

2. Example: Being a          Behavior/attitude:   a good listener
   good friend              Behavior/attitude:   _____

                           Behavior/attitude:   _____

3. _____         Behavior/attitude:   _____

                           Behavior/attitude:   _____

                           Behavior/attitude:   _____

4. _____         Behavior/attitude:   _____

                           Behavior/attitude:   _____

                           Behavior/attitude:   _____

5. _____         Behavior/attitude:   _____

                           Behavior/attitude:   _____

                           Behavior/attitude:   _____

You now have a plan that you can nurse into production. You have some ideas of where you want to go and what you want to do, and also the state of mind you need to accomplish your goals. Great job! It is important to maintain the integrity of your plan. No shortcuts and no selling your soul for gain are allowed. Otherwise, this will not work. I know it and you know it.

## What Symbol Will You Go By?

One of the most effective ways to make sure you keep your new life path always in mind, especially if you find yourself slipping away from it, is to assign a symbol to the type of person you want to be, one that you can quickly remember during times of struggle. Years ago and even today, groups of people have used symbols to represent their virtues and power. Some Native American families represent their clans with animal names, such as the turtle clan or deer clan, to show respect for their identity. Sports teams use symbols of power to represent themselves, such as bears and eagles. The symbols they choose give them a connection to a power icon and remind them of their connection to its attributes.

There are many such symbols, and it might be useful to select one that serves your purposes. You might want to consider the universal animal symbols. Having studied healing symbols for many years, I will share some of the popular descriptions of the power interpretations that have been ascribed to them. What symbol best represents who you aspire to be?

- **Wolf**—Although the wolf has gotten bad press for eating up young children or little puppies, the wolf spirit is honored as the symbol for family cohesiveness. Its nature is to have roles within the den, nurturing the pups by different wolves with a role assigned to each of them. They are also known for teamwork in their hunting strategies.

- **Eagle**—Used by many countries and clans, it is known for its height of flying and visionary qualities. The eagle spirit is also considered to be able to talk to God and convey plans and needs for a people.

- **Snake**—For generations, the snake has been noted for its power to heal through its venom. For example, the yellow snake (not extinct) was used in Greek temples for its mild venom and the increased ability to have healing visions. It also has the power to go down into the earth and converse with nature divinities, bringing messages to those on top of the land. There is the obvious reference and more onerous implications to the story of the Garden of Eden.

- **Bull**—The bull is a favorite among the Spanish cultures, probably because it figures into so many romantic tales. In most of the world, the bull is regarded as the warrior for its majestic pride and individualistic determinism. The symbol seems to shout, "I am mighty and fear no one." The horns of the bull have been a common feature of leaders worldwide, maybe for the same reason.

• **Deer**—The symbol of the deer is probably best known as a nurturing and gracious force. It's generous by nature with a sweet and nonaggressive stance.

• **Beaver**—As the premier builder, the beaver offers the symbolism of industrial energy and sharp focus. I could almost see the beaver in overalls and a hammer as he constructs a mighty home and expands into other realms. This is a symbol for someone who wants to get things done.

• **Turtle**—This is a creature that has survived millions of years with his home on his back. This is self-sufficiency at its best. No one can say this is not a powerful symbol, even if it is slow. Maybe that is not important if you consider longevity as the race.

• **Dragon**—The dragon has had bad press from all the Walt Disney portrayals of it as a monster. Its real virtue is as a protector of the castle or princess. Conjured of various parts of a snake, lion or tiger, fish, bird, and fire cannon, it has the many features that can be used for these reasons. It is loyal and brave.

- **Lion**—The king of the jungle and often the king of wisdom, the lion kills without malice. The act of victory is by gently suffocating its prey, not tearing and gutting like the tiger. Lions are not particularly aggressive, especially if they are not hunting for food. What I really like about the male lion is that when he gets old, his mates continue to support him by supporting his weight on both sides while walking him to his meals. That is power.

- **Horse**—The beauty of the horse seems to be its sleek, fast pace and its loyalty. It is strong and its energies can be harnessed. Together, the rider and steed can look as if they are one animal.

Symbols certainly are not limited to animals. Flowers and plants, insects like spiders, trees like the mighty oak, and even shapes like the circle, cross, and triangle are common symbols. You can blend your symbol with other dimensions, such as color. Ted created his power symbol as a red wolf, which he constructed as his characteristics of a good leader and teacher with high passion (red).

Consider which of these colors best represents you:

• **Red**—passionate, warrior-minded

• **Black**—mysterious, magical

• **White**—pure, honest

• **Purple**—spiritual, high-level thoughts

• **Brown**—basic needs, natural

• **Light blue**—happy, joyous

• **Dark blue**—deep joyful thoughts, useful insight

• **Light green**—youthful thoughts, optimistic

• **Dark green**—achievement, harvester

• **Yellow**—creative, intelligence

# A New Path

This chapter focused on the creative side of your personal journey. What tools would you take if you were going on a real journey and all you had at your disposal were natural elements? How much faith in yourself do you have to succeed without the security of a backup plan? How much courage would it take to go out on your own and do something new?

This is a new place for you to stand and take inventory of what you want to accomplish during the rest of your life. Your brain was battered and contaminated. Now it is free. You are free. Your brain has been reformed and is now able to give you the best efficiency you can have. You have a new opportunity to look ahead and determine a path you can freely take with peace of mind. Embrace this opportunity, and it will give you the power to confidently rejoin your community and the people you love and reset your internal compass for a life you will be proud to lead.

# CHAPTER SEVEN

# Step Six: Re-establishing Your Internal Compass

If you had known Joan before the event that caused her PTSD, you would not recognize her after the event. Even though she had regained her brain functions through hyperbaric chamber treatments and excellent vitamin supplements, she was a very bitter person. She could talk about her devastating experiences very clearly with you and would do so at every chance she could. She wanted to coordinate PTSD groups in order to tell the story of how she overcame the huge challenges, but in reality she had yet to do so.

Joan's story was horrific. She had been captured by enemy soldiers while serving as a nurse in Vietnam. From the first, she was a victim. The encounter was full of blood and guts as she attempted to help the soldiers who were dying. When her unit was overtaken, she had been brutally beaten and raped by three enemy soldiers. Stabbed in the stomach and left for dead, she endured severe pain and nearly died on her way to the hospital.

There was no question she endured severe challenges in forgiving the world for her fate, and she had lost a lot of her life to the problems of rehabilitation. PTSD had claimed almost twenty years of her life already; she was nineteen at the time of her capture. And it could claim the rest of her life unless she could reset her internal compass.

Joan reported that her previous life was a happy one, full of mischief and adventure. She had been a very popular high school coed, competing in beauty contests at the county fair. By age nineteen, she had married her high-school sweetheart (the captain of the football team), and had fulfilled a long-term goal of going to nursing school. She then joined the army medical branch as a way to see the world. So many of our military medical corps members, men and women alike, have endured horrific situations in the line of duty. Joan's experience may be among the most difficult to recover from, but I will tell you how it is possible.

Joan's story at this point serves to illustrate that her compass was pointed to *V* for *victim*. The world had misaligned her to a point of view that rearranged every experience to that perception. Men victimized her, her husband victimized her, everybody victimized her at some level, and here she was, soaking in all the tragedy that she had endured.

I will tell you the rest of Joan's story later, but when she saw me coming, and I challenged her with some changes that would reset her compass, she did not like me at all in the beginning. I became just another victimizer along her road to misery. It was true that she was treated horribly, and no one can or should erase that. But sooner or later we have to make a decision not to be victimized repeatedly. That is our decision and choice, and it is your next and final step on the road to full recovery from PTSD.

## Your Compass

A compass is an instrument that uses the Earth's polarity to keep pointing north. With a compass, you can always get your bearings regardless of where you are or what you see.

Think of your internal compass as the basic orientation to the world that keeps you focused. For most people, their internal compass keeps them pointed in a positive direction. If you are suffering from PTSD, your compass may be pointing in the wrong direction. For many people, it may still be pointed to *victim*. This chapter will help you rebalance your internal polarity so that you can find your own true north again.

You may find this chapter distressing because the goal is to turn your compass around from victim to a more positive direction. That fact is, if you have PTSD, you were somehow injured and possibly devastated by an event that was perpetrated by some other person, either intentionally or accidentally. And because of that fact you were defined as being a victim. You may be the victim of a war event, a rape, a terrible crash of some sort, or any number of horrible situations no person would choose. This set of events places you in the role of sufferer.

You, therefore, have a direct cause you can point to for your damages. And if you cannot find a resolution to these damages yourself, you can take it out on the world, right?

No. You instead need to have your internal compass reset to your true north. I realize that you were traumatized in some event that left you vulnerable and at least a little off track from your life plan. And it may not seem fair to ask you to leave that all behind, to have to take on the work of recovery when you didn't cause the problem in the first place. But when you get to the end of the line, you will find positives in taking on that change, and you are the only one who can do it.

If you are holding on to any thoughts and feelings about being a victim, you are probably experiencing heavy emotions now because you can't afford to use these thoughts as your compass any longer. They are eating your soul away and will eventually keep you fixed in a stage of permanent disappointment, anxiety, and fear.

You must know, though, that no one is accusing you of being a victim on purpose, or saying it is your fault. PTSD can happen to the navy captain who has eighteen years in the navy, including three wars, and a picture-perfect life, just as it can happen to the enlisted marine from the slums of an inner city, whose father was absent from his life and whose mother worked two jobs when he was growing up. It can happen to the trauma team doctor on the front lines as well as the chaplin, the special forces, the pilot, the helicopter gunner, the cop, or retired soldier turned military contractor who works to support our military operations.

But know that no matter what your situation—if you chose to volunteer for military service and ended up a victim of an explosion, torture, or a crash, or had some other life-altering event that may make you a victim—you too can have your internal compass reset to your true north. And just like Joan, this can take place decades after the event or the onset of PTSD.

Consider this process to be a positive phase of your life instead of categorizing it as merely a miserable one. Since we can't change the past, the hope is that we eventually see some of its blessings. And when we reset our compass, the blessings become much more clear.

## Does Your Compass Need to be Reset?

You may not know whether you have a need to reset your compass. The test below can help you. In the questionnaire below, I would like you to answer the questions as honestly as you can, even if you have to bear some guilt and resentments. Answer each with one of these responses: (A) for all of the time, (M) for most of the time, (S) for some of the time, and (N) for never or rarely.

1.  *I am very angry about the incident(s) that caused my PTSD.*
    (A)   (M)   (S)   (N)

2.  *I feel that somebody has to pay in order for justice to be served for what happened to me.*
    (A)   (M)   (S)   (N)

3.  *I feel bitter about the events and nothing has been resolved justly.*
    (A)   (M)   (S)   (N)

4.  *I find myself thinking about seeking revenge for the injuries done to me on the person or people responsible.*
    (A)   (M)   (S)   (N)

5.  *I find it almost impossible not to tell my story whenever I can.*
    (A)     (M)     (S)     (N)

6.  *I think that my whole life has been ruined because of the incident.*
    (A)     (M)     (S)     (N)

7.  *I think that if the incident(s) did not happen, I would be totally happy and free from worry now.*
    (A)     (M)     (S)     (N)

8.  *I cannot get on with my life because of what happened to me.*
    (A)     (M)     (S)     (N)

9.  *No one will have me now that I am damaged goods.*
    (A)     (M)     (S)     (N)

10. *I am always wondering, "Why me?"*
    (A)     (M)     (S)     (N)

Scoring: Count three points for every time you marked an (A), two points for every (M), and one point for every (S). Add all of the item responses for a score in a range from zero to thirty.

- 21–30: You have not let go of the PTSD and need to focus on letting these issues resolve at another level. That is the purpose of this book, to offer a menu of ways to get to a higher level.

- 5–20: You are fighting yourself and are fixated on revenge or resolution, making yourself vulnerable to disease and depression.

- 0–4: You have made great progress in moving on with your life.

If you scored a five or more, the following sections can help you reset your compass and build and rediscover the blessings in life.

## Getting Back Your Humanity and Rituals

If you find that you have cynical attitudes about humanity and the inherent goodness of life, try using a ritual to reconnect with these feelings. Humans have used rituals throughout time to mark the stages of our development. Rituals show that we honor the process and enable us to cope better with those challenges that are so troublesome. They include birthdays, holidays such as Christmas and Hanukkah, and special celebrations for accomplishments, such as graduations and marriages. We also have rituals to honor people for who they are or what they have contributed to our lives, such as awards and recognitions. Some rituals are for those times we need support from our family and community and for recognition of our progress. Those are the kinds of rituals we will explore in this chapter.

These types of rituals have three parts: a beginning, middle, and ending. Typically the beginning is a symbol of where you are in your stage or in the problem that needs to be resolved. For example, you may wear old clothes that you will discard as a sign of releasing the old fears, or announce that you will eventually change your old name to one that is free of emotional garbage. For example, if your name is Betty, but your aunt Betty was a drunk and your cousin bullied you by that name, you might feel relief with a new name you choose.

The middle is the process in which you transition to what you will become. The last phase is when you demonstrate the change you want the community to see. This phase is often accompanied by supportive behavior from the community and gifts for the future.

## The Ritual of Finding Your Mission in Life

There are many different rituals you can use to reset your compass, and those rituals may be a part of your current or past life. I won't attempt to cover them all in this chapter; I trust that if a ritual in your life brings healing to you then you will have the strength to pursue it. But, for anyone who does not have a ritual on hand to pursue, I will offer one example that I have seen have positive results for victims of PTSD.

In this example, you will work through the ritual of seeking to know your mission in life. It is called a Vision Quest ritual. Aspects of this ritual come from Native American tribal and European Celtic rituals that have served many people well.

The Vision Quest ritual is especially relevant for PTSD patients because it is a step forward into the future after releasing the emotional burdens of the past. If your brain is rattled, you probably need a way to rediscover yourself and where you belong in the big picture. There is no doubt that we are all connected in some way, that what we do with our lives affects one another, that we are all part of something greater than ourselves. (We even know from the laws of physics that when we unite together there is much more energy to make things happen.) We focus on solving problems together with a united intelligence. And perhaps we are all part of God's plan, and you are to play a part for total humanity. It is within this bigger plan that we play out our lives. And as long as we know our roles, we stay united with each other. This process is not necessarily religious, but conversely does not violate the edicts of any religion. It is a process of personal discovery that acknowledges the role of the universe and all things in it, seen and unseen.

In the Vision Quest ritual, the first step is to announce that you will be finding out your vision for your mission in life. To prepare for the process, you will need to dress in a ceremonial way. This is a specially created garment prepared just for this process. You create whatever brings meaning to you. It could mean using your mother's old scarf because of her protective ways and wearing two different shoes to symbolize their place in two or more worlds of understanding.

The second part of the ritual is a very dedicated process. You need to plan for it in order to be successful. Pick a place—it can be anywhere, such as your closet or a hotel room, although I think it works in nature best (I prefer the desert). You need to plan to spend as many as seven days and nights alone in this place, where only one person will come and check on you to see if you are OK.

You can bring a canteen of water, to be replenished by a friend if need be. No cell phones, iPods, or any other man-made distractions. You are to use the time to listen only. You are to stay within your drawn circle regardless of weather conditions (which makes it interesting). You have to be committed to doing this ritual right.

You are on the lookout for a vision that will give you your life mission. This ritual is to last seven days, but your vision usually comes in three days or fewer. In fact, many visions occur within the first hour, because once the distractions are gone, your mind moves fast. It has been waiting for this for a long time.

The mission will come, usually in the form of a symbol that will appear in your consciousness. (We'll discuss how to get that process started in the following section.) The message might appear in several forms until you finally get it.

In the case of Joan, she thought she saw a pencil, but when she went to examine the object, she saw that it was actually a twig. Then she daydreamed of an eagle, which startled her, but she could not understand what it meant. Then she dreamed of her mother, whom she respected all her life. As she pondered these three things, she saw a coyote looking at her that seemed to be posturing by standing one way and then another, always looking at her.

The coyote had marks where it had been injured. Then she came to a realization: the coyote was symbolizing herself and showing her life signs, but she had to be an example of success rather than a victim. Her mission was to step up and be a success for her family and community. She was to make herself beautiful so people would see how powerful she had become. And she was to write about her mission.

As she exclaimed her mission aloud, she felt relief. Although she had only been conducting her ritual on a ranch for two days, she was filled with energy and excitement. As a symbol of her mission for all to see, she bought a charm of a goddess and wore it as a necklace.

As the last part of her ritual, she announced her mission to her family and friends in a poem:

I am not the first, nor the last to suffer humiliation.
Nor will I be written about in books in days ahead to be
     bought.
But it is my mission for my family and loved ones to see,
That my soul will continue to soar and by Satan will not
     be caught.

I will step up to this path that has been ridden little,
And spread my wings of glory to share with my teacher and
     guide.
The awesome majesty of human spirit and power God has
     given
That my children will look to with hope and a lot of pride.

Then she brought forth the necklace and showed it to everyone, describing the symbolism of each facet and putting it around her neck.

Now it is your turn. The first part is to ask the universe, in a prayerlike fashion, to give you your mission and quest. You can say these words or merely acknowledge them with a yes to the question of your intent. The real effort is in the preparation for your next phase, the location and equipment you will need. I made a preparatory sheet below so you can fill it in as you go:

Intention or announcement of goal:

_____

Location of ritual:

_____

Preparation materials:

_____

_____

_____

Remember, once you start the quest, you cannot go back for more things. You are to remain in your place until the answer is known and you can take the next step. Ultimately, the goal is to realize the idea that you are part of something bigger than yourself and have a role in the journey of life.

Once you have settled yourself in the place of your mission journey, it is time to clear your mind of distractions. This will be difficult, because we live in a sea of distractions, and many are worries that lie dormant until we have enough silence to hear them. There may be layers of distractions that come from the past. *Is Uncle Bill doing OK? I haven't called him in months, and I promised him I would. Oh, I wonder if I turned the heater off in the bathroom. I hope Jennie or Susie is doing all right. Etc., etc.*

The key is to calm your mind and allow it to go through all the tangents it needs so all the worries, anxieties, fears, schedules, and other clutter clear from your mind. It might be good to remind ourselves of the calming effects good long breaths can have on the body and mind. When this is done, you will be able to listen more intently. That is the reason we close our eyes and bow our heads when we pray. We have to shut out the noise. As you clear your mind, start listening and looking both outside and inside your head. Use the following sheet to take notes if you need to.

Successful ways I have found to clear distractions:

_____

_____

_____

_____

Things that I see and observe that happen more than once or seem remarkable:

_____

_____

_____

_____

Things or messages I hear or receive that happen more than once or seem remarkable:

_____

_____

_____

_____

_____

Ideas and conclusions about my mission and where I am to be a part of something greater than myself:

_____

_____

_____

The rest is easy. When you have found a clue and something you can verbalize, you just pick up your stuff, give thanks to the universe, and leave. You can express your ideas to anyone you wish. It can be a party, or it can be a conversation. But it is important to tell at least one person. This makes it real. To leave it in your head unexpressed leaves it mushy and unarticulated.

## Becoming the Messenger

Once you have achieved your ritual and reset your compass, you may think your journey is done. This is not the full truth. In order to fully go forth with your new life path, you must become a messenger and bring this message of recovery to others.

The act of becoming a messenger is also a ritual and can be as subtle as being kind to another person or offering a smile to a frightened individual. Or it can be bold, such as offering directions in life, assuring a person of his or her ultimate success, or forgiving a person of a grievance. It's an important step in switching your compass from stagnant victimhood to a more positive direction. You may be doing this already, but if not, focus on becoming a messenger of hope and graciousness for someone else.

Forgiveness, toward those that caused the traumatic event or anyone else who has caused pain in your life, can be an especially tough but powerful action for those who suffer from PTSD. This kind of action can be a huge step for you. It is so powerful that there should be centers devoted just to the spiritual side of healing and forgiveness. Some find this in churches, and in fact I believe there is a spiritual component to healing and forgiving that is too often overlooked by many in the healing professions out of fear of mingling with religion. There is a wholeness that we all seek in the healing journey and that can only occur if we include the spiritual aspects.

A recent guest on *Dr. Phil* described her experience with

forgiveness on the show: "Forgiveness is like a whole new life philosophy for me. It is almost like a religion with me now. The peace I achieve when I truly forgive someone who has hurt me is as peaceful a place as I have ever been. I carry this thought with me always: *Forgiveness does not overlook the deed. It rises above it.*"

She is right. Forgiveness is not forgetting. It is not condoning or excusing the event, saying that whatever happened was OK, because it was not and is not. It is not letting people escape accountability and responsibility for what they did. Forgiveness is releasing that issue of hate and revenge to something else. And I can assure you that we all have consequences for our deeds. I have seen hundreds of times how this comes about. Eventually justice wins out and balance returns to the world. That is a promise, and it is represented in our physical world in an infinite number of ways.

There are hundreds of opportunities each day to become a messenger of hope and graciousness to those around you. As you fulfill your ritual, you will likely become aware of the messages sent back to you. It might be a butterfly landing on your shoulder, a squirrel that says something in squirrel language to you, or the magical moment of witnessing a shooting star. I know I can always count on my dog's welcome when I come home. Dogs are angels in furry disguise, and I would offer one to every person in the grips of PTSD if

I could. Or it could be the dance of a piece of paper floating in the air as it is carried by air currents. These moments are characterized by a sense of peace and joy.

This is the direction that will give you the best of what your life has to offer, regardless of how cloudy or mixed up you are at the moment. Any experienced airplane pilot will tell you that you have to trust your instruments. You cannot make good judgments in the air if you can't trust your orientation. You will be in a tailspin within five minutes without your compass and related tools. You have to trust your compass when your life is on the line. Your mental compass, set correctly, will be what sets your mind and soul at peace.

# Finding Joy

There is one more ritual I would like you to consider, and it involves finding joy. One of the most significant effects of PTSD is losing the ability to find joy in life. After all, one of the natural ways we set our compasses is toward happiness. The ritual we'll discuss in this section may sound a bit challenging, but remember that joy is a personal value and is different for everyone.

Recall that PTSD can cause the pleasure centers in the front of your brain to essentially turn down to a very low level of activity. This makes it difficult for you to find your compass and discover the joy in your life. Without positive reinforcement, our brains don't have a clue as to how to get pleasure. In the past we may have loved to caress our children, but now without the pleasure center being activated due to PTSD, that doesn't work anymore. Or maybe we used to like to drink beer and watch football to achieve that joy, but now that doesn't work either.

This ritual involves finding that direction again, and may take some effort and trials. It may sound selfish, but it is the process we have to learn again in order to understand others' needs as well. It also sounds simple, and it is.

This ritual is simply to have a party for yourself. This can be a celebration party for being who you are or for some achievement you feel happy about. For example, I would like to have a celebration every time I mow the lawn. I hate mowing the lawn more than getting a tooth pulled, so I want some gratification every time I do it.

For you, it could be a celebration of something as simple as mowing the lawn, or it could also be as profound as beginning a journey or returning from a journey. I am sure some reason to celebrate yourself will come to mind.

The real effort is designing a party in celebration of you. First you must decide how many people and who to invite. Some people like a lot of people, some people like a few, and some don't want any. I am generally one of those strange individuals who has done my own celebrations by myself for so long, I like to have it that way. (I guess it is my style from being raised in a family that did not have parties, other than a few bridge parties my parents enjoyed.)

But this is your celebration, and some of your decisions to be made are below:

People to be invited: _____

Activities to be planned: _____

Place: _____

Reason given for party: _____

Food and drinks: _____

Gifts: _____

Music: _____

Entertainment: _____

I am sure there will be other things to work out, but just be sure you enjoy it. And if you don't, do it again with some modifications. The important thing is to learn to celebrate yourself in your own way and to learn joy without caution.

## Summary

This chapter may be the last "step" chapter, but it is not the final step in your life. It was intended as a guide to your next step in life. These steps are a bridge from one side of PTSD to the other, and will be instrumental in helping you through some obstacles to healing. If you are still struggling with some issues, you can go back for another try, because sometimes you might miss something the first time through.

Do not get discouraged if everything is not totally on an even keel. This does not mean you are too damaged to be helped. The goal is to give you a framework for hope and reset your compass for positivity and success.

There are stages of changes, such as the ritual making and finding joy, that will give more honor to your process. The brain is developed to find happiness and avoid misery, but there are many ways people do this. Some use trial-and-error, some use logic. Some study them for a lifetime, some experience only once in a lifetime. But no matter which of those paths is right for you, the important thing to know is that there is help, and new directions that we have only begun to explore. And always remember the people who love you.

# Chapter Eight

# Forwarding Words

There are a number of exercises that can be done that may hasten your recovery from the ravages of PTSD, but the most important exercise is to love yourself and give allowance for the time it takes to heal. Regardless of how good you are or how powerful a person you see yourself as, time is the biggest healer of all if you can allow the next day to be different from the previous one. You have to be patient with yourself. It gets discouraging to see the sun set at the end of the day and feel no progress, but no one said things would be simple.

Much of this may feel like you take one step forward and move three steps back. There are sure to be ups and downs, but the most important thing to remember is to simply not give up. This is a practice that you will get better and better at, but at times, although you are making progress, it may feel as if you are not. Stick to it, and you will surely see results in time. After all, you don't run the Marine Corps marathon without first learning to run one mile and then five miles and so on.

There is no such thing as a PTSD recovery plan for everyone. Even though the program in this book is designed to be broad enough to work for everyone, the reality is that each person is different. There will be some aspects that work well for you and others that will be less important. But in whole, the methods do work. You will discover your own path, and I want you to constantly remind yourself and everyone around you about your progress. We are all growing.

There will be a strength that grows within you from all your experiences. As they say, if it doesn't kill you, it will only make you stronger. That is the way of the body and mind. There is no secret to how people have grown through pain and suffering. Always know that you are special, and that is why you have survived.

## Talk to Yourself

There is one more method I would like to leave you with before we conclude. Try this in the privacy of your home or car because it requires you to talk aloud to yourself.

It may sound a bit odd, but repeating words aloud to yourself is another aspect of brain plasticity as well as self-care. Studies have shown that when children talk to themselves while trying to solve math problems, they find the solutions easier. In fact, all types of learning increase when you can vocalize the process. To varying degrees, we are all visual and auditory learners. By saying something out loud, we are helping the brain in two ways: the exercise of saying something and the process of hearing and processing what we have heard.

Thus, it will be helpful in your journey to find some consoling words or mottos to repeat aloud to yourself when you are alone, such as:

- I know I can.
- I know that I am blessed.
- I know I am loved.
- I know I will.
- I know I will be OK.
- There is a place for me.
- This too shall pass.
- The only time I lose is when I quit trying.
- Success is a decision, not a destination.
- I am here for a reason.

Repeat these to yourself often, and you will see results you never expected but that are supported by science.

It makes sense that what is happening can be justified scientifically. Brain maps show that repeating phases will begin to modify your brain in such a way as to integrate the message you are conveying to yourself. People who meditate report that if they don't repeat their mantras every day, they get restless and unsettled. There is a peace of mind and resolution to higher self-esteem that occurs when a person repeats a personal motivational phrase one thousand times a day.

It might be the rhythmic sounds you are making with your tongue that influence the frequency of the brain. Or it could be the act of speaking that stimulates more blood to the brain. But no matter why it works, repeating a positive mantra such as the ones mentioned previously can bring you close to a life of love, where PTSD is only a memory.

## Loving Yourself: Lesson 101

Another important thought to leave you with is that you are loved. Loving yourself is not selfish but supportive of the truth: you are beloved. There is someone who cares what happens to you, I am sure. Maybe it is your mother, maybe a sister or brother. Maybe it is your spouse or even someone you don't know exists.

I remember Nell who came into our clinic with a terrible set of problems, all of which were tied to being abused, raped, and neglected by her family. She told stories about how her mother would continue to berate her for anything she did. This was all the more amazing, and heartbreaking, because of the things Nell attempted on her own behalf. For example, she wrote a song that was actually published and sung by her high-school choir, not because she was an honorable student but because it was really a beautiful song. In spite of this achievement, her mother actually convinced her that she did not write the song because she was not that smart. Nell finally agreed and never picked up a pen again, even though she had many songs in her head.

As we worked at the various techniques, I remarked that I noticed there were many people who were watching her with respect for how brave she was. She was totally taken aback by this remark, and I thought I might have made her paranoid, because she wanted to know who said this and where they said it. Finally we agreed to do an experiment. We decided that she would start wearing a small scarf around her neck, in a fifties, Doris Day style. We would see how many people would notice.

The following week she came in with such a look that I could not tell if she was amazed, embarrassed, or just surprised. Her eyes were wide open, and she had trouble explaining herself through her excitement. She reported that many of the girls at her church started wearing the scarves, small girls she did not even know. When she inquired to the mothers (whom she did know), they reported that the girls were trying to be like her because she was their hero. As it turned out, a lot of her friends knew her story (from high school and other sources) and had reported their admiration to their children.

Nell felt strange, being in a new role that was beyond her normal experience. And the change was magic. Being a role model, she had to be more than she thought she could be. She felt responsible for modeling the "right stuff." This experience had to be balanced with a sense of being genuine to herself, but the change in attitude was remarkable. At last her story could serve as a better message that the victim she had been had become a hero who overcame adversity.

And that is the principle that I am asking you to think about. You are not alone. You have a friend, and one of your best friends is you. So be good to yourself. You may just be a hero to someone else.

## Can You Do It by Yourself?

Perhaps one of the most important things to remember is that you can't achieve this recovery by yourself. Many people feel they need to do everything by themselves, because that was the way they were raised. I felt this way too. When you are out in the middle of the country and the fence is broken or the tractor won't run, there is no one else. But I had my knees kicked out from under me on more than one occasion by this attitude.

I remember one time in my career when I was suffering tremendously from a pain syndrome that might have left me paralyzed for life. I had a young family to support, and I had lost my job. My unofficial adoptive mother came to me with some good advice. She told me that it was time to ask others to help me, especially those who cared for me, because that was a way of loving them. People like to do things for people they love, and I was depriving them of that if I pushed them back. I was staggered by this revelation. This struck me at my core of beliefs, but she was right.

There are times when you have to ask for help, but that doesn't mean you are weak. It means that you are allowing love to come in as well as go out. And amazingly, my pain problems went away, and I learned the most important thing in my life: I didn't get that job back, but I didn't really want it after all.

I still find it hard to ask for help; I won't lie. But I do believe in the power of love. I also believe that it is mostly our egos that sabotage us from success in life, and we are really meant to be part of something bigger that gives us the power to overcome these challenges. The first step in twelve-step programs is to become aware that you are incapable of managing your life by yourself. I believe that is also true for the challenges of PTSD.

I do believe in your strength and your success, and if you need to ask for help, why not? The acquired power is always to your advantage. And who doesn't need some extra love? I never turn that down.

You can always use another person or source on your team, especially if you get the help you pray for from the big guy up there. I am always surprised where some of the most profound directions come from. It might come from that silly cousin, who suddenly comes up with a great line that resonates with you. Or maybe even a dog that inspires the right step.

There is luck in the world, and I think it rewards you when you commit yourself to a supreme mission. It is funny how things work that way. When you make the effort to set a plan, and put the work in to follow that plan, things seem to come out better than you ever could have planned.

I believe in the Compass RESET Program, I believe in your plan, and I believe in you.

# Stress Reduction Script

Reduction of stress is perhaps the most important medicinal thing that we can do for ourselves—for our bodies, for our minds, and for our own sense of who we are. When we don't get the right quality of restoration, we suffer physically, psychologically, and perhaps even spiritually.

I want to offer these steps for you to find the skills to reduce stress and carry it into the middle of your life. So let's begin.

It is hard to read and relax at the same time, so I recommend that you either have someone you trust read the recommendations to you with a gentle voice, or that you read them into a recorder and then listen to the recording.

*First, get yourself into a very comfortable position. Often people are in uncomfortable positions, so they literally have to hold parts of their body up. It is very important for you to find a position in which you can completely relax on a physical basis. Most people either lie down or sit in a very supportive chair. Next, just begin to let things go. Let go of your plans for tomorrow or next week. Let go of what has already happened, such as your reactions to an argument, confusion on the job, or another part of your life you want to come to some sort of conclusion. This needs to be let go. This needs to be put out of your mind for the time being. Remember this is not the time to problem solve or find solutions. This is the time to let go. This is also the time to let go of worries. This may be difficult for you. But it's important to do so to allow some kind of mechanism to release your worries. This is a choice. To worry is a choice of your mind and how to use it. So please make the choice not to use your mind to solve the worries that you have right now. It's not a time to worry about money, not even a time to worry about health. Let your soul allow your mind to be supported and to feel safe. Imagine putting all your worries about your family, your job, etc., into a bag or a box and handing it over to someone else. Someone in your mind. Perhaps a spiritual being. Perhaps someone like God or a special person in your life, to take care of them for the time being. Allow your mind to trust this being, to trust the world, to trust the universe. You don't have to worry about these things right now.*

*So let's just practice this image for a few moments. First of all, imagine taking all of your worries and plucking them like you might pluck oranges. Plucking them out of your mind. Not that they are not important. Not that they don't deserve some attention. But not right now. Take them and put them in your worry box. Each one is very deliberate. Think of all your worries. Pluck them out of your mind. Put them in your worry box. And as you do so, you may just feel a sense of release. You may let out a breath of release. Ahhh, letting go. Some people may feel a little bit undeserving of allowing these worries to be taken away for even a short period of time. But this is important, and it's a choice of how you use your mind. It is very inefficient to keep these worries at this time. Put them in a basket or a box and give it to some other source. You may hide them, you may put them under the ocean, or you may give them to God. You may have a certain friend or angel to give them to and maintain them if you wish. Now allow them to go, allow them to disappear for the time being. Now all you have to do is surrender yourself to the needed sleep. Surrender your weariness, surrender your fatigue, and allow your body to sink down into this spot where you are now.*

*One of the most important features of learning to relax is learning to breathe. Your breath is a signal. The pattern of your breathing is a signal to the rest of your body so that you can begin to allow all of your systems to go into sleep mode. By breathing the relaxation pattern, your mind can shut down, your heart can actually begin to rest itself better. All of your organs, your kidneys, your lungs, your pancreas, your intestines, and your muscles can begin to relax as well. You no longer have to hold on to anything. Follow this pattern: breathe in and breathe out to about the same count. For example, breathe in to a count of seven—one, two, three, four, five, six, seven—and out—one, two, three, four, five, six, seven—and in—one, two, three, four, five, six, seven—and out—one, two, three, four, five, six, seven.*

*Now continue this same cycle, paying attention to your breath. Just paying attention to the breathing in and the breathing out at about the same pace. It may not be the seven count. It may be some other kind of pace. But it's the pace that's important, and I'm going to emphasize that over the next few moments. Of just breathing in and breathing out, breathing in and breathing out. In and out, in and out. Continue to breathe at an even pace. Just focus on your breathing, nothing else. In and out. Focus on that pace. Pay attention to how it feels when you breathe that air in and when you breathe that air out. When you breathe in, you're breathing in food for your body, you're breathing in inspiration, you're breathing in love, breathing in power. And when you are breathing out, you are letting go. You're letting go of things you need to let go of. You're letting go of toxicity, physical toxicity, and mental toxicity, poisons, used-up air, used-up resources. It's important to breathe out all those things. You're cleansing, cleansing your mind. And this is what relaxation accomplishes, a cleansing. Letting go of things you need to let go of. The cycle of breath is a way of cleansing your body. The relaxation cycle is a way of making your body and your mind healthier and healthier. In order to get on with life, we need to allow those things that we need to discard to be discarded. Breathing in and breathing out. Perhaps feeling cleaner inside. Feeling more refreshed, and most important, feeling more peaceful. Breathing in and breathing out. Allowing that peace to enter in. To enter that sense of safety, security. This is the time that you will be protected by many wonderful sources. Please be assured of that as you breathe in and breathe out and allow your breaths to take you deeper and deeper into relaxation. Deeper and deeper into letting go. Deeper and deeper into surrendering any worry that may stress you. Surrendering to the basic source from where we came. Just breathing and relaxing more and more. In and out, taking you deeper and deeper into relaxation.*

*And as you are breathing and relaxing, let us focus on your feet. Your feet have been carrying you all day. They are very strong, but they need to be relaxed. So as you are breathing, sur-render any kind of tension or stress in your feet. Allow them to be bathed in comfort and in peace. Breathing in and breathing out, you may even notice they become warmer. You may have a sense of tingling in your toes. Very good, excellent. Breathing in and breathing out. Allow your feet to relax. Surrender any kind of tension in your feet. Allow that concentration to go up into your lower legs, your calf muscles. And again allow those muscles to relax. Just breathing in and breathing out, that peaceful cycle. And your legs will begin to relax automatically. Allow that sense of comfort to be relaxed and released with each breath. Now bring that attention to your upper legs, to those powerful muscles in your thighs and in your hips. Again using the relaxation cycle of your breathing to relax them more and more. And to relax any kind of tension you may have in those areas. Allow those muscles to become more and more relaxed, flaccid, and trusting. Your muscles can be trusted to relax and can trust the support you have. Maintain any kind of posture, any kind of defense. They can truly relax and feel safe. Breathing in and breathing out. Having that sense of security. Bringing your attention up into your stomach, where you often hold most of your anxiety and your stress. When you can, let go of those butterflies in your stomach. And you do this by your breath. Allow your stomach to rise and fall and allow all that jitteriness, the unsafe feelings, the insecurities, to just go out with your breath, and replace it with a wonderful sense of peace.*

*Breathing in and breathing out. Allow this part of your body to become part of the whole. Just relaxing, allowing those things you need to let go of, those insecurities that have been building up, to just go away with your breath. And perhaps as well you might feel a sense of warmth in your stomach. This is good. Breathing in and breathing out. Feeling the love. Reach down into your stomach, a sense of worthiness, a sense of peace. Breathing in and breathing out. You might even experience a sense of joy because of the understanding you might have with the peacefulness. A new profound peace. As you accept this comfort. As you accept the security, breathing in and breathing out. Feeling the renewal of your body and your mind going into your chest. Your chest encapsulates your heart, the passion, and also the pain. The pain of rejection, the pain of self-criticism. Let those go, let those go through your breath. Cleanse your heart, cleanse your chest. Feel a sense of caring. Feel a sense of support, a sense of perhaps even specialness. Just breathing in and breathing out. Very good! Excellent! Breathing in and breathing out. More and more relaxation. Deeper and deeper into relaxation and sleep. Breathing in and breathing out. Feeling as if you are being held and comforted. Perhaps even rocked, rocked into sleep. Feeling that sense of wonder about yourself. And accepting that kind of gift. There is no reason to reason this out. There is no explanation for this sense of support. It is just a gift. Accept it with each breath. And now focus on your shoulders. Your shoulders are the most frequent sources of stress. Because we hold so much responsibility on ourselves. We have to deal with the burdens of the daily work. This is the time to shed those responsibilities and allow yourself to be lighter, to be freer with each breath. Breathing in and breathing out. Allowing your shoulders to let go. Let go of the burden. You don't have to carry any burden right now. You can let that go with your breathing pattern. Breathing in and breathing out.*

*And allowing that relaxation, that deep relaxation to enter into your shoulders and to go down each arm. Relaxing each muscle and letting go. Down into your hands. Your hands that carry so much responsibility, that do so many things, so many tasks. Allow them to relax. Allow them to experience your breathing cycle. Become more and more relaxed. Deeper and deeper into relaxation with each breath. Very good. In and out, allowing your hands to relax. Become warmer, become more peaceful. Breathing in and out. In and out, letting go.*

*Going up through your neck and inside your head. Relaxing the muscles inside your head as well as around your head. Using your breathing to relax the muscles around your ears. Around your jaw. We often hold anger in our jaw. We want to speak out. There is no need to do that right now, just relax your jaw. Breathing in and breathing out, relax your jaw more and more. Very important part of your body to learn how to relax. Breathing in and breathing out. Moving deeper and deeper into relaxation. Into the sleep cycle that you deserve. Breathing in and breathing out. Relax those muscles behind your eyes. Those six main muscles you can relax with your breathing. In and out, relaxing. Relaxing over the top of your head. There are big flat muscles that can be relaxed. These are often muscles that can cause stress headaches. It's time to relax those muscles with your breathing. Allow those muscles to become twice as relaxed, twice as relaxed with each breath. With each breath becoming more and more relaxed, deeper and deeper into safety. Letting go of those tension spots all over your head. Especially coming from your neck over the top of your head.*

*And as you are breathing, allow your whole body to expand and contract with your breath. You will know when you are totally relaxed because your whole body can expand and contract. There is a certain plasticity that occurs. Enjoy that sense of relaxation. Keep in mind that even if you are not in deep sleep by now, you are in a state of relaxation that is equal to sleep. So maintain this relaxation, don't become frustrated with yourself. Allow yourself to surrender. To surrender to whatever you need to surrender to.*

*As you relax feel free to continue the relaxed state for the rest of the day. You have completed the relaxation script. Please be aware that there are no demands to be continued through this relaxation script that would be binding for the future, just the awareness that relaxation is good for you and can be integrated into your day.*

*Whenever you wish, feel free to get up and go about your day, whenever you wish, knowing that your body and mind are restored. Go with many blessings...*

# Resources

ADAA. (2007). "2007 Stress & Anxiety Disorders Study." *Anxiety Disorders of America.*

Aftanas, L. and Golosheykin, S. (2005). Impact of regular meditation practice on EEG activity at rest and during evoked negative emotions. *International Journal of Neuroscience,* 115(6), 893–909.

Allman, J. M., Hakeem, A., Erwin, J. M., Nimchinsky, E., and Hof, P. (2001). The anterior cingulate cortex. The evolution of an interface between emotion and cognition. *Annual New York Academy of Science,* 935, 107–117.

Amir, S., Brown, Z. W., and Amit, Z. (1980). The role of endorphins in stress: evidence and speculations. *Neuroscience Biobehavior Review,* 4(1), 77–86.

Ancharuff, M.R., J. I. Munroe, and Fischer, L. M. (1998). "The Legacy of Combat Trauma." *Internal Handbook* of *Multigenerational Legacies of Trauma* ed. Y. Daniel. Plenum: New York, 257–275

Biederman, J., Wilens, T., Mick, E., Milberger, S., Spencer, T. J., and Faraone, S. V. (1995). Psychoactive substance use disorders in adults with attention deficit hyperactivity disorder (ADHD): effects of ADHD and psychiatric comorbidity. *American Journal of Psychiatry*, 152(11), 1652–1658.

Bittman, B., Berk, L., Shannon, M., Sharaf, M., Westengard, J., Guegler, K. J., et al. (2005). Recreational music-making modulates the human stress response: a preliminary individualized gene expression strategy. *Medical Science Monitor*, 11(2), BR31–40.

Carmody, J. and Baer, R. A. (2007). Relationships between mindfulness practice and levels of mindfulness, medical and psychological symptoms and well-being in a mindfulness-based stress reduction program. *Journal of Behavior Medicine*.

Cartwright, D. (2002). The narcissistic exoskeleton: the defensive organization of the rage-type murderer. *Bulletin Menninger Clinic*, 66(1), 1–18.

Chapell, M. S. (1994). Inner speech and respiration: toward a possible mechanism of stress reduction. *Perceptor Motor Skills*, 79(2), 803–811.

Christie, W. and Moore, C. (2005). The impact of humor on

patients with cancer. *Clinical Journal of Oncology Nursing*, 9(2), 211–218.

Department of Veteran Affairs HSE&D (August 2009.) *The Assessment and Treatment of Individuals with History of Traumatic Brain Injury and Post-Traumatic Stress Disorder: A systematic Review of the Evidence.*

Doidge, N. (2007). *The Brain that changes itself*, Penguin: New York.

Eriksson, P.S., Perfilieva, E., Bjork-Eriksson, T., Alborn, A., Nordborg, C., Peterson, D. A., and Gage, F. H. (1998). Neurogenesis in the Adult hippocampus, *Nature Medicine*, 4 (11): 1313–17

Esch, T., Duckstein, J., Welke, J., and Braun, V. (2007). Mind/body techniques for physiological and psychological stress reduction: Stress management via Tai Chi training—a pilot study. *Medical Science Monitor, 13*(11), CR488-497.

Flora, S. J. (2007). Role of free radicals and antioxidants in health and disease. *Cellular Molecular Biology (Noisy-le-grand), 53*(1), 1–2.

Foote, B., Smolin, Y., Neft, D. I., and Lipschitz, D. (2008). Dissociative disorders and suicidality in psychiatric out-patients. *Journal of Nervous and Mental Disorders, 196*(1), 29–36.

Frisman, L. K. and Griffin-Fennell, F. (2009) Commentary:

Suicide and Incarcerated Veterans—Don't Wait for the Numbers. *Journal of the American Academy of Psychiatry and the Law.* 37 (1): 92–94.

Grafman, J. and Litvan, I., (1999) Evidence for four forms of neuroplasticity. In J. Grafman and Y. Christen (eds.) *Neuronal plasticity: Building a bridge from the laboratory to the clinic*, Berlin: Springer-Verlag, 131–39.

Grafman, J. (2000) Conceptualizing functional neuroplasticity. *Journal of Communication Disorders*, 33 (4) 345–56.

Hanover, J. L., Huang, Z., Tonegawa, S., and Stryker, M. P. (1999) Brain-deprived neurotrophic factor overexpression induces precocious critical period in mouse visual cortex. *Journal of Neuroscience*, 19: RC40:1–5.

Harch, P. G., Fogarty, E. F., Staab, P. K., and Meter, K. V. (2009) Low pressure hyperbaric oxygen therapy and SPECT brain imaging in the treatment of blast-induced chronic traumatic brain injury and post traumatic stress disorder. *Cases Journal*, 2:6538: 1–4.

Hiem, C. and Nemeroff, C. B., (2009) Neurobiology of Posttraumatic Stress Disorder. *The International Journal of Neuropsychiatric Medicine.* 14 (1): 13–24.

Hoge, C. W., McGurk, D., Thomas, J. L., Cox, A. L., Engel, C. C., and Castro, C. A. (2009) Mild Traumatic Brain Injury in U.S. soldiers returning from Iraq. *The New England Journal of Medicine.* 358: 453–463.

Huang, Z. J., Kirkwood, A., Pizzorusson, T., Porciatti, V., Morales, B., Bear, M. F., Maffei, L., and Tonegawa (1999) BDNF regulates the maturation of inhibition and the critical time of plasticity in mouse visual cortex, *Cell*, 98:739–55.

Institute of medicine of the National Academies (2009) Gulf War and Health: Long term consequences of traumatic brain injury. 7 Washington: The National Academics Press.

Ippolito, C. J. (2007) Battlefield TBI: Blast and Aftermath. *Psychiatric Times*. 3 (8).

Jacobs, B. L., van Praag, H. and Gage, F. H. (2000) Depression and the birth and death of brain cells. *American Scientist*, 88 (4): 340–46.

Kennedy, J. E., Jaffee, M. S., and Leskin, G. A. (2007) Posttraumatic stress disorder and posttraumatic stress-like symptoms and mild traumatic brain injury. *Journal of Rehabilitation Research Development*. 44: 895–920.

King, N.S. (2008) PTSD and traumatic brain injury: Folklore and fact? *Brain Injury* 22: 1–5.

Kjellgren, A., Bood, S. A., Axelsson, K., Norlander, T., and Saatcioglu, F. (2007). Wellness through a comprehensive Yogic breathing program—A controlled pilot trial. *BMC Complementary and Alternative Medicine, 7*(1), 43.

Kolb, B. and Whishaw, I. Q. (2003) *Fundamentals of Human Neuropsychology*, 5th Ed. Worth Publishers: New York.

Krauss, M. R., Russell, R. K., Powers, T. E., & Li, Y. (2006). Accession standards for attention-deficit/hyperactivity disorder: a survival analysis of military recruits, 1995–2000. *Military Medicine, 171*(2), 99–102.

Johnstone, J., Gunkelman, J., and Lunt J. (2005) Clinical database development: characterization of EEG phenotypes, *Clinical EEG Neuroscience.* Apr;36(2):99–107

Labbe, E., Schmidt, N., Babin, J., and Pharr, M. (2007). Coping with stress: the effectiveness of different types of music. *Applications in Psychophysiology Biofeedback, 32*(3–4), 163–168.

Lawlis, F. (2009). Re*training your brain*, Plume: New York.

Lutz, A., Greischar, L. L., Rawlings, N. B., Ricard, M., and Davidson, R. J. (2004). Long-term meditators self-induce high-amplitude gamma synchrony during mental practice. *Processings National Academy of Science U S A, 101*(46), 16369–16373.

Neri, S., Signorelli, S. S., Torrisi, B., Pulvirenti, D., Mauceri, B., Abate, G., et al. (2005). Effects of antioxidant supplementation on postprandial oxidative stress and endothelial dysfunction: a single-blind, 15-day clinical trial in patients with untreated type 2 diabetes, subjects with impaired glucose tolerance, and healthy controls. *Clinical Therapy, 27*(11), 1764–1773.

NINDS. (2002). National Institute of Neurological Disorders

& Stroke Post-Stroke Fact Sheet. *The National Institute's of Health National Institute of Neurological Disorders and Stroke, NIH Publication No. 02–4846.*

Office of the Secretary of Defense SBIR 2009.3—Topic OSD09-H08 Title: *Early Detection of Mild Traumatic Brain Injury.*

Sapolsky, R.M. (1996). Why stress is bad for your brain. *Science,* 273 (5276): 749–50.

Schwartz, J. and Begley, S. (2002) *The Mind and The Brain,* Harper-Collins:New York.

Sherman, C. (2007). The defining features of drug intoxication and addiction can be traced to disruptions in cell-to-cell signaling. *NIDA Notes: National Institutes of Health, National Institute of Drug Abuse, 21*(4).

Taniellian T., Jaycox, L. H. (Eds). (2008). *Invisible Wounds of War: Psychological and Cognitive Injuries.* Center for Military Health Policy Research, the Rand Corporation, Arlington, VA.

Tarazi, F. and Schetz, J. (2005). *Neurological and Psychiatric Disorders,* Humana Press: New Jersey.

Tikkanen, R., Holi, M., Lindberg, N., and Virkkunen, M. (2007). Tridimensional Personality Questionnaire data on alcoholic violent offenders: specific connections to severe impulsive cluster B personality disorders and violent criminality. *BMC Psychiatry, 7,* 36.

Van Praag, H., Schinder, A. F., Christie, B. R., Toni, N., Palmer, T. D., and Gage, F. H. (2002) Functional neurogenesis in the adult hippocampus, *Nature Neuroscience*, 5 (50): 438–45.

van Stegeren, A. H., Wolf, O. T., Everaerd, W., and Rombouts, S. A. (2008). Interaction of endogenous cortisol and noradrenaline in the human amygdala. *Progress in Brain Research, 167,* 263–268.

Wang, X., Merzenich, M. M., Sameshima, S., and Jenkins, W.M. (1995) Remodeling of hand representation in adult cortex determined by timing of tactile stimulation. *Nature*, 378 (6552): 71–75.

Wildmann, J., Kruger, A., Schmole, M., Niemann, J., and Matthaei, H. (1986). Increase of circulating beta-endorphin-like immunoreactivity correlates with the change in feeling of pleasantness after running. *Life Science, 38*(11), 997–1003.

# About the Author

Dr. Frank Lawlis is a renowned psychologist, researcher, and counselor with more than thirty-five years' experience. He is a fellow of the American Psychological Association. Dr. Lawlis is the cofounder of the Lawlis Peavey PsychoNeuroPlasticity (PNP) Center and is the chief content advisor for *Dr. Phil* and *The Doctors*. He is the author of more than one hundred articles and several books, including *The ADD Answer* and *The IQ Answer*. He is a contributing blogger for *Psychology Today*.

# Index